Raising a
TEAM
PLAYER

Raising a
TEAM
PLAYER

Teaching kids lasting values
on the field, on the court,
and on the bench

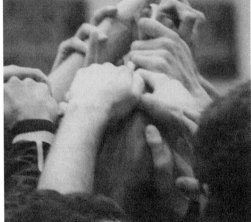

HARRY SHEEHY
with Danny Peary

STOREY
BOOKS
North Adams, Massachusetts

*The mission of Storey Publishing is to serve our customers
by publishing practical information that encourages personal
independence in harmony with the environment.*

■ ■ ■

Edited by Nancy W. Ringer
Art direction and cover design by Wendy Palitz
Cover photograph by Giles Prett
Photo credits appear on page 152
Text design by Laurie Baker
Layout and production by Susan Bernier and Cynthia McFarland

Copyright © 2002 by Harry C. Sheehy III

The information in this book is true and complete to the best of our knowledge. All recommendations are made without guarantee on the part of the author or Storey Publishing. The author and publisher disclaim any liability in connection with the use of this information. For additional information please contact Storey Books, 210 MASS MoCA Way, North Adams, MA 01247.

Storey Books are available for special premium and promotional uses and for customized editions. For further information, please call Storey's Custom Publishing Department at 1-800-793-9396.

Jacket printed in the United States by John P. Pow Co.
Printed and bound in the United States by Quebecor World
10 9 8 7 6 5 4 3 2 1

Library of Congress Cataloging-in-Publication Data

Sheehy, Harry.
  Raising a team player: teaching kids lasting values on the field, on the court, and on the bench / by Harry Sheehy with Danny Peary.
    p. cm.
  ISBN 1-58017-447-7 (alk. paper)
  1. Sports for children—Coaching. 2. Sportsmanship. 3. Conduct of life.
I. Title: Teaching kids lasting values on the field, on the court, and on the bench.
II. Peary, Danny, 1949– . III. Title.
  GV709.24 .S54   2002
  796'.083—dc21   2001057640

DEDICATION

To Mom,
who taught me to laugh every day.

To Dad,
who taught me that the applause of a single
human being is of great consequence.

And to Connie,
whose faith, balance, and perspective
are a constant source of inspiration.

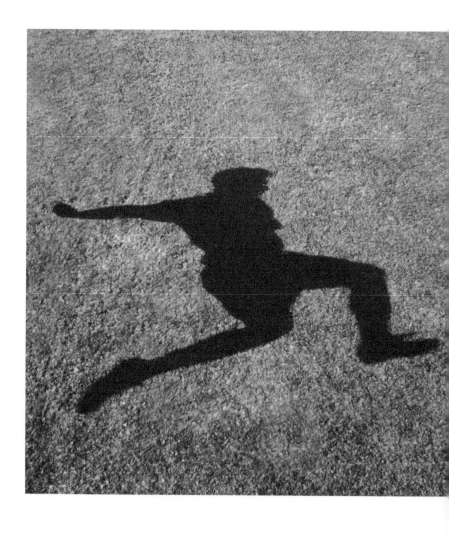

CONTENTS

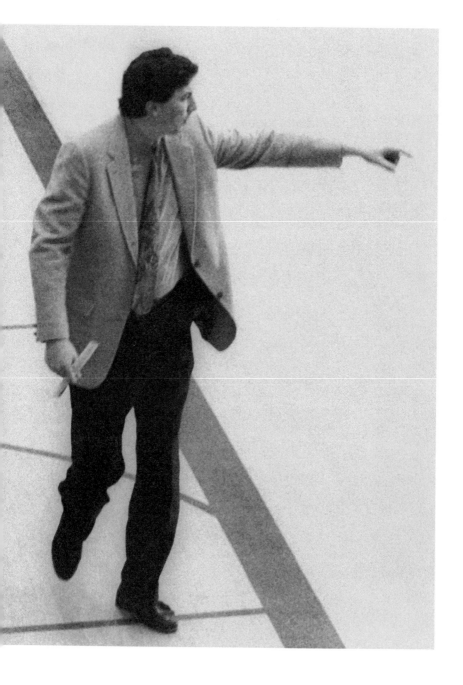

ACKNOWLEDGMENTS

I FIRST STARTED THINKING ABOUT THIS BOOK YEARS AGO, BUT the idea finally came to fruition thanks to the people at Storey Books. Without their belief in the need for *Raising a Team Player*, the undertaking never would have gotten off the ground. My co-author Danny Peary and I are most grateful to our editor, Nancy Ringer, who provided patience, guidance, and a firm hand when necessary to move the project forward. We also wish to acknowledge the support and enthusiasm we received from publisher Janet Harris, editorial director Deborah Balmuth, creative director Wendy Palitz, designer Laurie Baker, art director Cindy McFarland, graphic designers Erin Lincourt and Susan Bernier, photo coordinator Laurie Figary, and publicist Stephanie Taylor. We are grateful to have worked with a team who all want to raise team players. We also want to express deep gratitude to Melissa Kay Rogers, Jennifer Unter, Karen Ware, Robert Rosen, Caroline Schechter, Maury Gostfrand, Gail Lockhart, Barbara Hadzicosmas, Suzanne Rafer, and Laura Peary. And many thanks to Yankees manager Joe Torre for contributing the foreword.

I have been fortunate to have many people influence my life through sports in a positive manner. John Bardong, my Little League baseball coach, not only taught me the game but also showed me that good teaching and fun can go hand in hand. My junior high coaches Richie Smith, Bob Allen, and Con Chigger constantly emphasized fair play and sportsmanship. I don't think any young athlete could have been coached by better people.

During my seventeen years as the men's basketball coach at Williams College, my players demonstrated work ethic, sportsmanship, competitive spirit, and enthusiasm on a daily basis. My sincere thanks goes out to all "my guys," who inspired me far more than I ever could have motivated them.

The most important team in my life is my family. Thanks to Mom for rewarming countless dinners because I was at the park playing until the last glimmer of light faded. I have wonderful memories of Dad and I traveling to countless games as I was growing up, and of his constant message: "The game is pure." I am grateful to still be taking these trips with Dad today. Finally, thanks to Connie, my bride of twenty-five years, whose beauty, poise, and faith are as irresistible today as when we first met over thirty years ago.

FOREWORD

WHEN A NEW YORK YANKEE WALKS INTO A ROOM, PEOPLE WILL say, "Wow, you're a member of the New York Yankees!" They don't say, "Wow, what's it like to play with Derek Jeter? What about Bernie Williams and Roger Clemens?" This is fitting because, I am proud to point out, on the Yankees, the team is always more important than the individual players, and the statistic that matters most to my twenty-five players is the number of world championships we've won. We have been able to lure big-name players like Jason Giambi and Mike Mussina to New York because, despite having had tremendous individual success, they coveted the opportunity to play on a world championship team. Having captured four World Series titles in six years, the Yankees are regarded as winners, and when new guys walk into our clubhouse, they seem to want to fit in with the way we do things. They are after a ring of their own, proof that they were part of the best team in baseball.

In this insightful, challenging, and much-needed book, Harry Sheehy expresses numerous ideas that are similar to my own, and I certainly agree with his view that winning, while a great goal, isn't everything, especially in amateur sports. Still, there is no doubt in my mind that winning as a team is much more significant and rewarding than having success as an individual. I wouldn't want to downplay personal accomplishments, but *winning as a team by doing all the right things well* should be every athlete's primary goal. This ideal should be taught much more often on the professional level; even more important, as Harry points out, it must be injected into youth, high school, and college sports.

Almost every professional athlete played in organized sports programs in their youth. Why have so many come through that experience without having developed good character traits, learned good sportsmanship, or discovered what it takes to be a winner, including sacrificing for the good of the team? Youth sports would seem to be ideal for introducing solid values to kids, but as Harry laments in this book, too few kids are allowed to have fun, enriching experiences. That's because many win-at-all-cost coaches and misguided parents fail to teach the proper lessons that kids can carry into their adult lives, whether they play professional sports or not.

Like Harry, I was fortunate. Sports was my saving grace as a youngster, too. I was immature and selfish and had my feelings hurt as much as anybody, and because I was overweight and had issues with a very critical father, I didn't like myself very much. But on the ballfield, where I had success and was part of a team, I felt differently. My older brother and idol Frank was a big leaguer, so I felt pressure to be a good example and not a bad sport. I also was lucky to have a sandlot coach, Jim McElroy, who impressed upon me that players should do whatever is necessary to help the team win, outside of breaking or bending the rules. I may have batted fourth in the lineup, but like all my teammates I'd be asked to squeeze bunt a run home to secure victory for my team. The fundamental lesson I learned, and that I now teach my players, is that for a team to win on a consistent basis, players need to exhibit unselfishness. I discovered that I could strike out four times and still feel good if the team won, as opposed to being happy if I got four hits in a loss.

My own philosophy includes many of the concepts I first learned as a kid playing for Coach McElroy; and what I teach major leaguers is appropriate for coaches to teach Little Leaguers. For instance, my players buy into the fact that winning as a team is more important than who the hero is. I point out that while big things, like 500-foot home runs and twenty strikeouts in a game, make the headlines, it's the little things that win ballgames. As Harry contends, if you string enough little things together, they spell *success*. Moreover, players are better able to concentrate because a big task like winning the game is never daunting if their focus is always only on little things like sacrifice bunting, running hard on the bases, and moving a runner to third base with less than two outs. In this way, they confidently leave things up to their teammates in certain situations, which means that when they win, it's as a team.

Everybody seems to be consumed with the bottom line — winning — yet hardly anyone is really interested in how you get there. From my perspective, if you are going to win, talent isn't enough. Even in professional sports, there are many athletes who are extremely talented but lack direction and have a hard time focusing their talent and energy on the team approach. It really bothers me to see all the talk and taunting that goes on in sports, most visibly in football and basketball, by players who have to tell you how good they are; it seems to me that the only person they are trying to convince is themselves. When interviewed, they make a big point about how they want to win a championship, but few of them have the necessary patience and commitment to do it. Believe me: Doing it and talking about it are two entirely different things.

These self-serving players often put up better numbers without going all out than less-talented guys who give you an honest effort, but when the tough times come, they aren't able to get the job done nearly as well. As the New York Yankees have proven since 1996, nothing is more important than the quality of the people involved. There is so much character inside players of high quality that isn't necessarily God-given. In most cases, it was learned and developed in their formative years, while they were involved in youth sports. The unselfish, forthright, principled players we admire and hold up as models to our young people — I would guess that they were the ones lucky enough to have someone teach them what it truly means to be a winner.

I have always judged people on effort as opposed to the bottom line, and I wish all coaches at all levels did the same. I think that if you go out there and make the maximum effort without being afraid to fail, you are a winner, no matter what's on the scoreboard. In 2001, the Yankees reached the World Series and almost became champions again even though we didn't have our best team. We may have lost in the end, but we showed what not quitting is all about — and that is a sure sign of a winner. As I told my players, it's all right to be disappointed when you don't win, but don't let a loss keep you from being proud of the effort you put out.

All athletes should be told that they don't have to be on the winning team to be a winner. Baseball is a game of life. Even the most successful people don't succeed all the time. Everyone tastes defeat. I think the best lessons are learned when you are maneuvering past the potholes of life and learning to deal with failure and rejection. I believe that you will become a better person and accomplish more than if you had never experienced adversity. It's like running the marathon: You can run to a certain point, but then you hit that "wall," and it takes extra effort to break through it. I believe that, unfortunately, a lot of players in baseball and other sports, whether they are youngsters or older, simply play until they get tired or frustrated, and then they back off.

Sports is a place where you can find out what's important to you. Do you want to be the best you can be? Do you want to win the big game, or would you rather just have a good game yourself? If you want to win, if you want to go for the title, then you have to reach inside and find what it takes to keep you on course until the end. You have to challenge yourself to accomplish anything significant. How important is it to you, and how hard do you want to work?

Most people, including kids, aren't on winning teams. In my case, I went through a seventeen-year playing career in the majors and many years as a manager without winning. Trust me: When it's all said and done and you finally have accomplished your dream, you'll find that it was well worth the wait. However, to motivate a kid to stick with a sport when things aren't going well, a coach has to make him feel good about himself. It can be tough to have that kind of influence, because, as Harry writes, when a kid walks into the house after a game, the first thing his parents want to know is usually the score — and that takes him down a peg or two. As *Raising a Team Player* stresses, parents should encourage kids to enjoy themselves, not discourage them by making wins and losses the most important thing. I firmly believe that participation in a game is much more important than the result. That is what coaches and parents must make clear to kids. Because Harry Sheehy and I agree that whether you're a professional athlete or a seven-year-old, it all boils down to five simple words:

Do the best you can!

PREFACE

YOUTH SPORTS HAVE BECOME A PRESSURE COOKER OF EXPECTA-
tions. Parents scream abuse at players, coaches, and referees.
Coaches demand that their kids win, at any cost. Kids practice day and night. They face intense pressure to score, to
win, to succeed. But is this the measure of success we want
to impress upon our children?

I was a late bloomer — skinny, small, and, despite my
obsession with basketball, tragically short of skills until I hit
my sophomore year in high school. Then a miracle happened
— I grew. In fact, I grew so fast that my bones hurt; my
mother had me soak my ankles in a bucket of cold water
every night to ease the ache. My legs caught up with my feet,
my skills caught up with my legs, and suddenly I was a
pretty decent player.

I went on to become captain of my high school basketball team and, from there, captain of the basketball team at
Williams College in Williamstown, Massachusetts. I played
semi-professional ball for eight years after college, touring
the world and playing against such opponents as the
U.S.S.R. national team, the Yugoslavian Olympic team, and,

here at home, collegiate powerhouses like the University of Michigan and the University of Maryland. Afterward, I returned to Williams to coach the men's basketball team. I worked with college-age players all winter long, then ran camps for young girls and boys — from bold seven-year-olds to gawky fourteen-year-olds — all summer long. In 2000, after almost twenty years of coaching, I set aside my coaching hat and became the director of athletics at Williams.

I've had the great fortune to make my living in a realm for which I feel true passion: sports. Through sports, I've been inspired, tested, taught, and humbled. Most important, from the time I first held a ball to this very second as I write, I've grown as a person. Tomorrow, and the next day, and the next, I'm sure, I'll keep growing. It's the nature of sports to be a constant teacher. It places its participants — players, coaches, referees, and fans — in situations of stress, tosses in a measure of competitiveness and expectations, and sits back to see the true nature of people revealed. We learn a lot about ourselves then. When we don't like the way we act in a competitive situation, we know that it's time for us to change and mature.

I was lucky to be born in an age that valued sports for the natural joy of it, not for the trophies to be won or as a step in a plan to turn a kid into a million-dollar professional. Imagine if I had been born into the current generation of youngsters. My father would have enrolled skinny eight-year-old me in the local youth leagues. I'd be a benchwarmer, getting just a few minutes or a few innings of playing time every game. The all-star travel team would manage just fine without me, thank you. As I got a little older, my friends and I would pick one or two sports that we really wanted to play. Of course mine

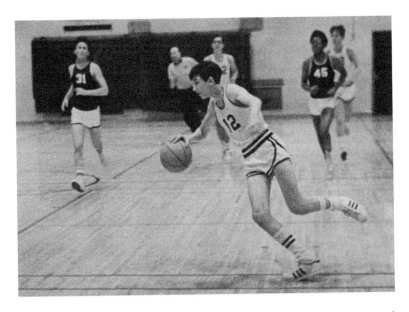

would be basketball, even though I still wasn't very good (that's me above, still small and awkward at fifteen). House-league coaches would push me harder and harder, anxious for me to perform at a better level. Other parents would groan and complain when I got out on the floor. "Win! Win! Win!" would be the constant cry, and knowing that I was not con-tributing — that I was, in fact, holding the team back — at some point I would become completely discouraged and quit.

If that had been the case, what would I be doing now? I don't know. All I can say for sure is that my life would be completely different. And I probably would not have had the opportunities — to be tested, to mature as an individual, to work in a field that I love, to travel the world, to work with young people — that my current life has given me.

What's happening in youth sports today is simply unac-ceptable. We place huge performance expectations on kids.

We ask and allow them at an earlier and earlier age to specialize in just one sport, ostensibly so that they can focus their skills and become the best player they can be. Think about it — even if every kid became the best player he or she could be, only a fraction of a percentage of them would ever go on to play professional sports. Why, then, do we place such huge pressure on them to win, to star, to succeed? Many kids with less natural talent are forced out of sports before they've had time to absorb the valuable lessons sports offers. And the kids who have enough talent to stick with the games — what sort of lessons are they learning? That

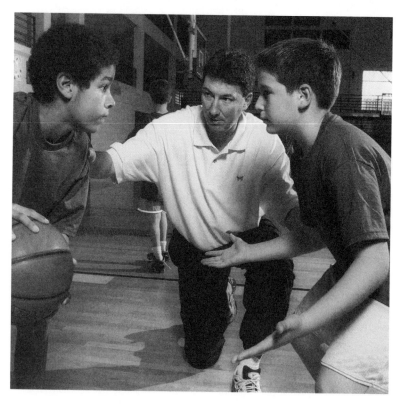

they must always win, at any cost? That their worth is determined by the number of points they can score? That sports is more important than school, friends, and family?

It has to stop. And the people who have the real power to stop it are parents.

Most parents understand — and lament — that standing on the sideline with a hat that says "Coach" doesn't make you a coach. They also know that having kids doesn't make you a parent. Parenting is a thought-provoking, time-consuming, and extremely challenging art. Today, most kids are hyperorganized, and parents spend their time running them around from one activity to the next. "Quality time" is limited to chatter in the car while you're driving to practice and a few mumbled words while the family is wolfing down dinner. With such hectic schedules, it can be difficult to find real teaching moments — those rare times when you, the parent, see a lesson that should be taught and your kid is in an open frame of mind and will actually hear what you have to say. Sports, approached in the *right way*, can be a gold mine of teaching moments. It offers parents opportunity after opportunity to have a positive impact on the lives and development of their children.

What is this "right way" to approach youth sports? Understand that:

1. Developing a strong value system is more important than winning.

2. Being a great team player is more important than being a great scorer.

3. The most important reason that kids play sports is because it's fun. When it stops being fun, they'll stop wanting to play, and they'll stop learning.

Why do you want your kid to play sports? Is it because you want him to develop a strong value system, learn to support and encourage his peers, gain self-confidence, and have fun? If your answer is yes, then you are on the right track, but you have a long uphill battle ahead, because that's not what most of youth sports today is about. We've built a system that is out of control. As a culture, we are consumed by our fascination with professional sports, and we have appropriated the winner-take-all attitude of paid professionals and misapplied it to our youngest athletes. Now coaches yell; parents demand; kids are tense, immature, and selfish. These attitudes don't belong in youth sports. You can't criticize a ten-year-old in the same way you criticize an adult. Nor can you expect her to have the same intensity, desire, and focus. For that ten-year-old, winning is important, yes, but even more important should be the pizza and party that come after the big game.

There's been a lot of press recently about the horrible acts of violence taking place in youth sports. Fans charge the field and fight with players. Parents corner referees after games and attack them. In the now-famous incident that took place in Reading, Massachusetts, in 2001, two fathers fought in front of their sons and other parents after a hockey practice. One ended up dead; the other, in jail.

As a nation, we are at a crossroads. We recognize that there is something terribly wrong with youth sports, but we lack direction on how to resolve the problem. The first step, I firmly believe, is for each of us, individually, to step back and reevaluate our expectations for sports. Why do we think that playing sports is a valuable experience for young kids?

If the value is a spot on an all-star travel team, a college scholarship, or a championship trophy, then we will act in a certain way to achieve those things. If the value lies in helping kids have fun while they learn to handle themselves in high-pressure situations and develop work ethic, passion, humility, excellence, character, and good sportsmanship, then clearly we will act differently.

We have lost a generation of young athletes to our misguided sense of values. Let's not lose another. Let's think differently. Let's act differently. Alone, this book will not be of great help; it is my hope that it will provoke new thoughts and new conversations. What's most important, parents, is that you get out there and get involved — in the right way. You are the ones who will make a difference.

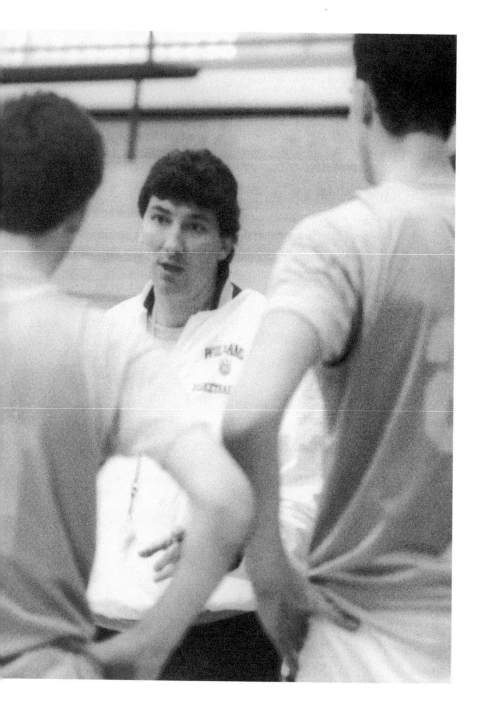

INTRODUCTION

During my seventeen years of coaching boys and girls at sports camps and the young men on the varsity basketball team at Williams College, some of the people who inspired me most in my work were my elderly acquaintances. What really struck me about them was that they hadn't retired from life but were still learning. I remember my late friend John Woodland, an English professor at Trinity Western University in Langley, B.C., whose belief was, "If I decide I have 'finished' learning, the truth is that I'm just discouraged, because there's always more to discover and experience." Even when he was sick and could no longer get around, John's mind remained active, and he wrote poetry and continued to educate himself. He still considered himself a work in progress. I thought, "If John was a work in progress at his age, then what about kids?"

Surely every young person is a work in progress, open to life lessons that will help them in their next steps of growth and maturity. Such learning takes place at home and in the classroom, but I don't believe that is sufficient. From the experiences of my own youth, I know that kids in their formative years will, under the *right* circumstances, benefit greatly from participation in sports.

Sports can stretch and grow kids. It can trouble and excite them. Frustrate and inspire them. Help them look deep inside themselves and open their minds to the world around them. Most important, sports can infuse young players with character and confidence that together will serve them for the rest of their lives.

◼ ◼ ◼

THE GOOD NEWS IS THAT THIS SHOULD BE THE GREATEST TIME EVER for kids who are involved in sports. Across the country, there are an increasing number of opportunities in camps, youth leagues, schools, and colleges for students to play every sport imaginable, at every age and skill level. So, in theory, the great majority of young people should be having tremendous fun playing games and improving their skills. But the bad news is that something has gone wrong. Many kids feel such stress and discouragement from pressure-filled experiences that they want to quit their sports entirely. Others are adrift, playing sports but having no understanding of what they can get out of them if they set goals and work hard to reach them. Too many with real talent have neither a passion for playing the game correctly nor any regard for teammates, opponents, coaches, or fans. Some are witness to terrible scenes of violence — players fighting with each other, fans harrassing referees, parents assaulting coaches. It's absolutely horrifying.

The games — baseball, football, basketball, soccer, ice hockey, field hockey, volleyball, swimming, tennis, golf, track and field, and all the others — are as great and pure as ever. Yet I see that youth sports are becoming remarkably unwholesome, ugly, even corrupt — I'm sure you will remember the scandal over the pitcher in the 2001 Little League World Series whose birth certificate had been falsified. Unfortunately, the blame for the bad attitude and, in many cases, bad behavior of kids rests mostly on the shoulders of parents and coaches, the very people who contend they want kids to benefit from sports.

There are many adults — both parents and coaches — who are incredibly positive influences on young athletes. However, too many overzealous moms and dads and tyrannical coaches are turning off kids to sports by teaching them, through words and example, all the wrong lessons. It's come to such a point that rules are being created to govern not kids but adults, such as soccer league Silent Sundays, during which parents are forced to keep quiet. In the current state of affairs, that's not a bad idea; I've attended some youth-league games that made me want to flee the stands and go home because I couldn't put up with parents and coaches screaming at the kids. Is it any wonder that we're losing kids, even those who are very talented, from sports? If I were a kid and some other player's parent were yelling at me, I'd certainly think about quitting. And that is what is happening across America today.

Oddly, I first started thinking about writing this book fifteen years ago when I was invited to attend a local youth-league basketball game. I was shocked that the coaches and parents were constantly screaming at the ten-year-old players, the opposing coaches, and the fourteen-year-old referee. Everyone had arrived with good intentions, yet when the whistle blew to start the game, few adults in the gym seemed to know that they had a responsibility to the kids to behave properly. It was loud, abrasive, and alarming. In the intervening years, I might have given up on the idea of writing the book, but today such games have become commonplace. There is a real crisis in youth, high school, and college sports.

I lament the passing of a golden era when kids of all ages would grab a ball and go out into the street, vacant lot, or field and play past sundown. The games were pure; kids had fun; they made up their own rules; they made friends. Yet organized sports has its own merits: controlled learning, team play, adult involvement. I believe that kids in their formative years can learn much more about sports and life — and have fun and

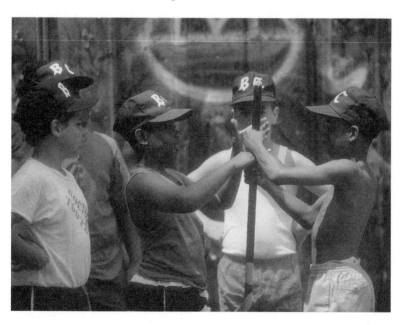

make friends in the process — when they are part of an organized sports program. That is, they can *if* they receive guidance from enlightened adults who are invested in both the improvement of their skills and the development of their characters.

Every young person will play a sport at some point, whether at school or in a youth league. This is fortunate, even convenient, for parents who want their kids to find themselves in situations that will stimulate their growth as individuals and as members of a team. Sports provides countless windows of opportunity for kids to learn moral, ethical, and character-building values. These are true teaching moments, and we should eagerly take advantage of them. It is my hope that *Raising a Team Player* will educate adults about what our kids need in order to have fulfilling, mind-opening sports experiences, and how they can help provide them.

■　■　■

IN THE REALM OF YOUTH ATHLETICS, THERE ARE THREE MAJOR players: the young athlete, the coach, and the parents. At the onset they must all ask themselves, "What about this game is important to me? What am I here for?" Sports will answer these questions; they will also help you translate those answers into terms that apply to the larger scope of your life.

Famed NBA coach Phil Jackson wisely said, "There's more to life than basketball, and there's more to basketball than basketball." I take it further: There's more to life than sports, and there's more to sports than sports. In addition to having fun playing a game, youngsters develop life skills. If through sports youngsters can have fun while discovering much about themselves, establishing a healthy lifestyle, and learning sportsmanship, humility, and self-discipline — particularly when they are very young — then it is incumbent upon us as adults to encourage our children to participate in sports. And we must be supportive. For the lessons we teach our children through athletics to have any impact, kids have to understand them and realize how they translate into the other parts of their lives.

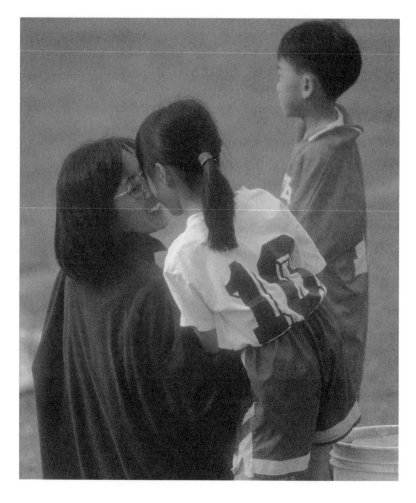

When athletes are young, all that is essential in sports is that they have fun. Kids who are six, seven, and eight years old are still learning how to use their bodies; half of them are completely uncoordinated — balls bounce up and hit them on their chins. But they have plenty of exuberance, and sports is an arena in which they can express and put to good use that natural joy in life.

As kids get older, what will separate them from the pack is skill. All skills can be taught. Of course, kids don't always need someone to take them by the hand and show them how to play the game; often they can work it out on their own. However, learning is made much more powerful for youngsters when they have adults supervising and encouraging their progress. Adult involvement can help kids develop more quickly — in their physical skills and in their emotional maturity — and it helps kids develop positive, strong relationships with the adults who are working with them. But even the best-intentioned parents and coaches often fail to recognize that there are more "acquired skills" than how to shoot a basketball, kick a soccer ball, hit a baseball, catch a football, spike a volleyball, or handle a baton pass. Excellence, competitiveness, humility, enthusiasm, being a great teammate, and other traits we want our young athletes to exhibit are also skills that can be taught and learned. Good, thoughtful coaches focus first on teaching such life skills. Thoughtless or inexperienced coaches may be so preoccupied with winning that parents have difficulty helping their kids see the good in the game.

I don't think there are many coaches who understand the scope of their influence. Maybe they want to coach a team simply because they like to coach; many coach because their kid is on the team. No matter what the reason, coaches must take the job seriously, because they are jumpstarting these kids in their athletic life, and all that it encompasses. How they handle the kids on their team — their own children and the other players — is *important*.

■　■　■

PARENTS SHOULD WANT THEIR KIDS TO BE INVOLVED IN A PROGRAM that is well run. For older kids, an athletic program is unique to their team or school. For younger kids, the program may encompass their entire league. Whatever the case, parents should expect a program to have clearly defined goals and core values. Ideally, these are written down and distributed to all players, coaches, and fans, whether as the program's mission statement or as guidelines for participation.

Good programs are so well established that when new kids come in, they adapt to the way things are done because they want to become part of something that is successful. We had a good basketball program at Williams, and I told almost every recruit, "You don't have to come here to create something good. It's been good for years. Your job is to create your own niche in something that is already good." That's a challenge for kids. One year, Matt Hunt, who was a Division III All-American for us, said in our highlight film, "The great thing about making the basketball team at Williams College is that as soon as you show up on campus, you learn how to act and how to be responsible to your teammates, coaches, and other students." A coach really knows he's had an impact when he hears his own players preaching the core values of the team. You've accomplished something; they're buying into your philosophy.

Although good coaches may downplay winning in favor of a good attitude, hard work, character, and enthusiasm, they still have to deal with outside pressures to win. The need to win to please outsiders who aren't interested in the personal development of the team's players is what makes a lot of coaches change their priorities for the worse. In fact, one reason I decided to stop coaching the men's varsity basketball team in favor of becoming the athletic director at Williams was that winning was becoming too important. Losing had never stolen the joy of the game from me, and I didn't want that to change.

If winning had become the most important goal of my basketball program, I would have let down the kids on the team. After four years, I wanted them to go off into the world having learned core values under my auspices, rather than believing that winning is the top priority. My guess is that they wouldn't ever call or come back to visit me if the main thing they learned was that losing is never acceptable. That's the wrong message to teach kids

A good coach puts as much effort into the lesson plan as any teacher. With luck, he or she will have passionate students who are eager to learn.

of any age. Every coach wants players who remember and respect him. Former players at the University of North Carolina would call and visit their former coach, Dean Smith, ten years after they played for him. They'd ask him for advice; they'd invite him to their weddings. When you invest in someone's life, as Smith did with many players, you have an impact that lasts. If you've just been coaching the game, and it's all

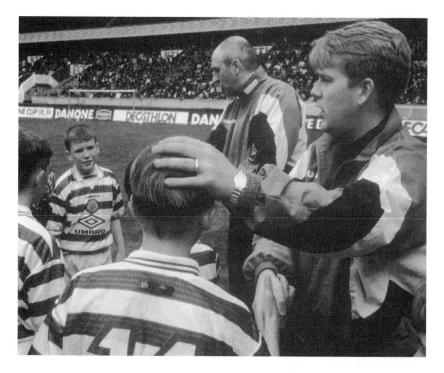

about winning and losing, then most players won't want to be a part of your life when the game ends. I am still in contact with my Little League coach John Bardong, who expertly taught us the game and made it clear that he also wanted us to have fun. I wonder how many players don't ever want to see their coaches again. I'm sure that happens more often than not, and that's quite sad.

I've noticed that many coaches screen for their kids the fact-based movie *Remember the Titans*. I must tell you that I am not sold on the no-nonsense football coach that Denzel Washington plays. I say this not because he used discipline to motivate his team, because that is essential to all sports teams, but because he used *questionable* discipline. I worry that this character is becoming a role model for coaches with a win-at-all-costs mentality. I prefer the warmer, though strict, basketball coach played by Gene Hackman in the fact-based *Hoosiers*. That coach used calculated, planned teaching to reach his high school kids. I believe it's important for kids to have planned teaching. The field, the court, the rink — whatever the playing arena, it is a classroom, and a good coach puts as much effort into the lesson plan as any teacher. With luck, he or she will have passionate students who are eager to learn.

■ ■ ■

IN YOUTH SPORTS, HIGH SCHOOL SPORTS, AND COLLEGE SPORTS, it's important that *everyone* understand that the game is only *part* of a student's life. The lives of professional athletes are consumed by the game, but that is not the case for student-athletes, nor should it be. At Williams, I had two hours a day to coach my players. I didn't want to have them in the gym five hours a day; they had school, families, a social life. Frankly, I'm shocked to hear how much some youth teams practice. They might play a game and have four or five lengthy practices during the span of a single week. What kind of signal does this send to youngsters who are just learning to put their priorities in order?

Though sports may have a huge impact on a child, as it did on me as a boy, it is a small piece of life, not all of it. I would always tell recruits, "I want you to choose Williams College as the place you would want to be if you injured your knee freshman year and could never play again. Then you're making the choice for the right reasons."

COACHES HAVE AN INCREDIBLE POTENTIAL TO AFFECT THE DEVELopment of young athletes. They serve as mentors and role models during the most formative, character-building years of a young person's life. My coaches changed my life. There was my father, Harry C. Sheehy Jr., who worked with me almost every day. I've already mentioned John Bardong; I still think of some of the things he said and the way he handled our team. I can say the same thing about Richie Smith, my ninth-grade baseball coach and the person who also happened to run the recreational program at the gym on Saturday mornings. I am also still grateful to Con Chigger, my junior high coach, and Bob Allen, who was a junior high gym teacher. All these people were my role models; they taught me the right things about sports and carried themselves like gentlemen in practices, in games, and in seemingly stressful situations.

There's more to sports than sports.

As role models, of course, parents are even more important than coaches. Psychologically and emotionally, they have the biggest impact on their kids. They also have the biggest challenge, for they are ultimately responsible for the character of their children. In the complex world of today's youth athletic programs, parents face a lot of questions. When is the right time to soothe a distraught child, and when is the right time to apply pressure? How do you encourage healthy competitiveness and discourage poor sportsmanship? How can you help your child develop a strong work ethic without letting him or her become discouraged at the slow progress? What's the best way to support a child who sits on the bench all year long? How can you encourage your strong-willed all-star to support his teammates? How do you teach a child to accept criticism positively? Most important, how do you help your child absorb real core values from sports? How can you use sports as a vehicle to talk to kids about life's challenges?

This book is intended to give parents insight into their kids' sports experiences: the right questions to ask, the right role to play, and the right attitude to model for their children. Parents, together with their children's coaches, have a hard job ahead of them. They need to praise, encourage, inspire, build, temper, support, and teach, working with their children on everything from setting goals to teaching sportsmanship and humility to building character and a sense of self-worth. All parents want their kids to learn these essential aspects of personal growth and maturity, and it's true that they can be taught to kids outside of the athletic arena. However, sports can be an incredible tool for teaching because it encourages learning in a way that sticks. The lessons you learn on the field, on the court, and on the bench — you remember them for the rest of your life. Our challenge is to change youth sports in America so that kids can have fun and learn these valuable skills, which set them on the path to a good life — the ultimate goal.

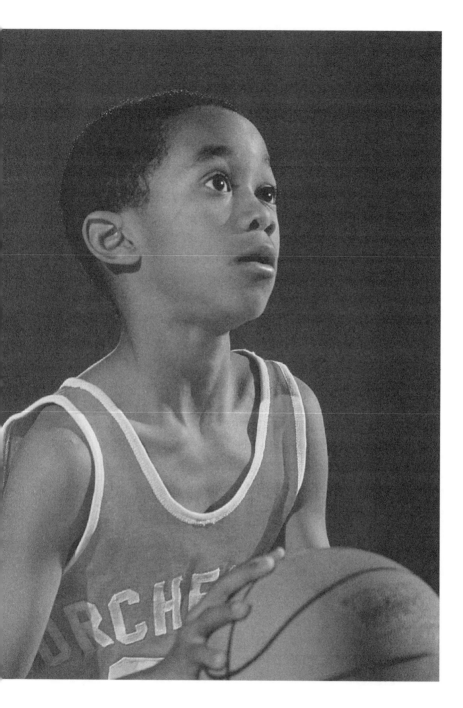

WORK ETHIC

My greatest joy as a coach was to teach kids who had so much passion for their sport that they were willing to work hard to get better. When I was recruiting high school seniors for my basketball team at Williams College, those were the kids I coveted. Quite often, beaming parents would come in with their sons and declare, "He loves basketball." But then I'd spend time with their boys and realize that they didn't love it at all. Mom and Dad may have seen Junior walking out the door with a basketball and assumed that he was working hard at the playground to improve his game. But he might have been the type to spend the day launching 25-foot hook shots and lazily walking after the ball. Or, if he had a baseball and a bat, he might have been interested only in seeing if he could reach the fences, swing after swing.

It's easy to mistake activity for passion. Anyone can participate in an activity, but without passion, a kid will not be motivated to work hard to become a better individual and team player. As a coach, I didn't want to recruit eighteen-year-olds whose parents or previous coaches hadn't already nurtured in them a passion for basketball and a work ethic to support it. I could enforce the rules of practice and make such players work hard, but would they have seen the inherent value of that work and adopted work ethic as one of their core values? By that age, it's usually too late. We develop our sense of character at a very young age, using the adults in our lives as models and mentors. If we don't learn a particular lesson when we're young, it's very difficult to learn it when we are older. That's why it's so important to start teaching values such as work ethic through youth athletic programs, while the kids are still young. Lessons learned early last a lifetime.

> *Games are won at practice.*

■ ■ ■

MOST GIRLS AND BOYS IN YOUTH, HIGH SCHOOL, AND COLLEGE sports understand that it's the coach's job to inspire them, but they don't understand that inspiration is a two-way street. They don't realize that we coaches — just like teachers — put out our best effort when our kids work hard enough to inspire us. What my best teams at Williams had in common was that they worked so hard to get better that I couldn't wait to get down to the gym each afternoon to teach them. Those young men, none of whom were there on an athletic scholarship, gave me an incredible effort every day, while also carrying full course loads and, with my encouragement, having active social lives. Because they inspired me, I'd often stay up past midnight studying film for them. And if any of them wanted to work on rebounding, shooting, or defense after practice, I made myself available.

I told my players, "Guys, I want you to work so hard that you feel in your heart that you deserve to win." That's *deserve* to win, not *will* win. You can't promise a kid that he'll always succeed if he works hard, but you can promise him that if he doesn't work hard, he will almost certainly fail. My challenge was to get my players to understand the need to work hard every day, not just on game day.

I have always believed that games are won at practice. Each of our twenty-four games was like an exam. How well had we learned the lessons undertaken in practice over the previous days? We "studied" such topics as "How Our Offense Can Solve a Zone Defense" and "What Makes a Man-to-Man Pressure Defense Effective." I drilled and drilled my players, because I would accept nothing less than for them to play hard on every possession. Many times we were victorious because our team was more fit than the opposition; we simply wore them out. Such success helped me sell this message: A work ethic is the foundation on which you build the goals that you equate with success. Every worthwhile accomplishment, in sports and in life, is made possible by a strong work ethic.

■ ■ ■

I AM LIVING PROOF THAT A STRONG WORK ETHIC CAN PRODUCE good results. After all, I'd been a young boy with no discernible talents but a willingness to work hard, and I went on to play varsity basketball at Williams and then to play for years with Athletes-in-Action, one of the top amateur teams in the world. When anyone asks how I became so adamant about the value of a work ethic, I say, "Let me tell you about my friend Brian."

Brian and I grew up together on Long Island. By the sixth grade, he was already 6'2" and brawny, and — no kidding — with a heavy beard at five o'clock. I was just under 5', slight, and definitely without a beard. We both loved basketball and played for our school's team. I was small and not very good, and when the game started, my job was to walk over to the corner of the gym and keep score on a chalkboard. Brian was so big that he overpowered everyone, and he was the star of the team. I went to practice every day and worked hard, but I didn't play more than two minutes in a game all year long. But I was fortunate. My father, Harry Sheehy Jr., who had played and coached both basketball and baseball, continued to encourage me. So rather than quitting, as many youngsters are apt to do when they aren't supported by coaches or parents, I went to work that summer to improve my game.

I asked my father to devise a workout plan for me. Then every day, without exception, I walked the twenty blocks to a small park that had hoops and worked hard on my game for a couple of hours. Meanwhile, my good friend Brian went to the beach. Every day.

In the fall, Brian and I both made the seventh grade team. Brian was still bigger and stronger than everyone else and was the best scorer and rebounder in the entire league. I went to practice every day and worked hard, but I still sat on the bench, despite having made some improvements. That next summer, and the following summer, too, I continued my workout plan at the park, and Brian continued to go to the beach. When it was 90 degrees and muggy and I was working, working, working, I thought of Brian at the beach, enjoying the sun and the sand, and I was envious.

I vividly recall the scorching day when my father came down to see how I was doing. It was about three o'clock in the afternoon, and the blacktop court was radiating heat. I just wanted to put down my ball and go to the pool or even join Brian at the beach. When my father was ready to leave, I said, "Dad, hold on. I'll take five more shots and go home with you." But that didn't sit well with him, and he gave me some advice he'd heard from Bill Bradley, who was then a Princeton basketball star and would someday become a United States senator: "Why don't you work ten more minutes," my father said, in a tone that made it clear his words were less a question than an order. "When Bradley was ready to quit his workouts, he always continued for ten more minutes because someone, somewhere else, had stopped. He figured that if he worked ten minutes extra every day, he'd win the contest between them if they ever competed." Dad's words made sense, and from that day on, first as a player and then as a coach, I always have said at the end of a day: "When you're ready to quit, work just ten more minutes. Work ten more minutes because someone, somewhere else, is quitting."

A work ethic is the foundation on which you build the goals that you equate with success.

Ten minutes may not sound like much, but multiply ten minutes by hundreds of practices. How much progress could you make if you worked just that much more?

I believe those ten extra minutes that summer paid dividends, because that fall I made the freshman team at Garden City High School. I was still small — I tipped the scales at a mere

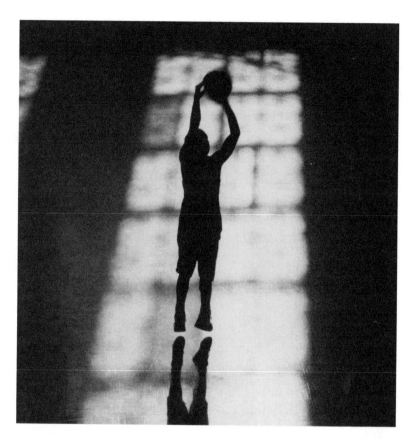

90 pounds and didn't crack the 5-foot barrier until halfway through ninth grade — but I could see my skills were improving, the result of countless hours spent on the court. Brian was still the star, but I actually got to play a little. And a lot of the other guys were starting to catch up with Brian physically.

By the tenth grade, I had grown a little, and my skills had started to sharpen to the point where I made the varsity team. Brian stayed on the junior varsity team. In the eleventh grade, we both made the varsity team, but I was a starter and Brian sat the bench. From beach to bench. After all those years, all those hot summers when I worked and he went to the beach, our roles had flip-flopped. Halfway through the year, he quit the team, frustrated that everyone was better than he was.

As I told my players, Brian was clearly good enough, strong enough, and skilled enough at an early age to have gone on to become a standout high school player. But he was already so much better than everyone else that he never thought he had to work on improving his skills. When everyone caught up to him physically, skills became the divider. By the eleventh grade, it was several years too late to start working hard.

No kid should be complacent about his or her skill level. Instead, as demonstrated by Cal Ripken Jr., the Baltimore Orioles shortstop famed for playing a record-setting 2,632 consecutive games, you must work every day to improve rather than have your skills diminish. And if you're big when young, you had better pay extra attention to skills because most kids who are big at an early age don't end up being 7 feet tall. Brian was 6'2" in sixth grade and never grew another inch. I was 5 feet tall and ended up 6'5" with skills.

Young players who see success early may think, "I'm already the best. Why do I need to be better?" Unless their coaches or parents encourage them, they see no need to work hard. But when you're not working, someone else is. And sooner or later, the two of you will come face to face.

■ ■ ■

SOME PEOPLE ARE INCREDIBLE ATHLETES, WHILE OTHERS HAVE NOT one speck of athletic ability. Most people, however, fall somewhere in the middle, and eventually it's skill that separates them. That's where work ethic becomes so important. I believe that work ethic itself should be considered a talent. It helps many athletes — Larry Bird immediately comes to mind — overcome shortcomings in other skills, such as lack of quickness and speed. And work ethic is a talent that carries over into all other areas of life. You may hear a kid say of another student, "She got an A on that test, but she isn't that smart. She just works hard." Well, that's a skill! It should be commended.

Ready to quit? Work just ten more minutes . . . because someone, somewhere else, is quitting.

Our children often hear from their peers that it's not "cool" to work hard. So it is imperative that parents and coaches show children — through their words, actions, and examples — that the ability to work hard is a fantastic talent to have. The earlier you can impress this upon a child, the better.

Of course, hard work for young kids isn't the same as it is for high school and college athletes. Coaching eight-, nine-, and ten-year-olds should be about encouraging passion for the sport, not about weeding out kids who aren't as good as the others. You want to help the eight-year-old understand why he has to work harder, but you don't want to turn him off to the game. Passion and excitement come first. Work ethic will follow.

Sometimes parents — who, as working adults, are accustomed to measuring the value of performance, not effort — are overbearing. But you must understand that if your nine-year-old is just a benchwarmer on a school or youth team, this doesn't mean that he won't become a terrific college player in that sport. It also doesn't mean that he won't enjoy and learn from his experience on the team. Some parents might say, "Well, if my child is not good enough to play on an all-star team in youth football, I will take him out of that sport and have him play soccer instead." If my parents had thought that way, I never would have played college basketball. I would have been pushed into another sport instead of being encouraged to work harder and realize my potential in the sport I loved.

I am gravely concerned by the earlier and earlier ages at which we expect results — victories, awards, trophies, and so on — from our children. What are the values we really want to teach? If there is not an encouraging adult around, be it a parent or a coach, to make kids understand what hard work and core values are, the sport they are playing may lose them before they have the chance to grow physically and develop their skills. We lose kids in the classroom, in music, in dance — everywhere — for the same reason. If they aren't taught with patience, enthusiasm, and the understanding that work ethic counts just as much as natural talent, the late bloomers will never bloom.

Too often, youth athletic programs are seen as a vehicle for getting children into college. We often overlook their true purpose: to provide kids with an opportunity to have fun while also building character and learning a number of lessons that will benefit them in every aspect of life. That's why some parents insist, "My boy should play," and blame the coach who doesn't agree. Wouldn't it be more helpful to the child if his parents said to the coach, "My kid needs a positive sports experience, and I really don't care how much you play him. He'll be at every practice, and he'll work hard." And wouldn't it be great for the youngster, when he came home, if his parents didn't say in one breath, "Did you win? That coach who doesn't like you — did he finally play you?" What if, instead, they said, "It's great that you're part of the team. Work hard so you'll be ready when you get a chance." Parents often believe that their child will become upset and disheartened if he doesn't get much playing time, and they think this is unfair. But they should understand that whatever role on the team the youngster's hard work creates is valuable, even if he's a substitute. It's a fact: For the majority of players, hard work will lead to a role on their team, not All-City, All-State, or All-American status.

If a player works hard only because he thinks he can become a star, he's doing it for the wrong reason. Some day, somewhere, some time, he'll be disappointed with his achievements. He'll end up saying, "Well, I think I should be starting, and my dad thinks I should be starting. But Coach won't start me, so I don't think it's worth working so hard anymore." But if that player has developed a work ethic, he will understand the value of working every day. He will find that it helps him at every turn, in every challenge, for his entire life.

One player who found his niche on my team at Williams College was a young man named Seth Mehr. He had been on the junior varsity team as a freshman and tried out for the varsity the next year. My assistant coach said, "You've got to cut him." But I liked that he had a ball with him all the time, and that when I'd go up to the gym, I'd find him there working endlessly. Finally I said, "You know, I believe there is a role for a kid who works that hard." Seth created a role for himself; his hard work convinced me to keep him. In time, he became the captain of a team that went to the Division III Sweet Sixteen, and he played 10 to 12 minutes a game. He made a real contribution in practice and in games. After graduation, Seth went on to medical school and became a doctor. He wrote me once to say, "Coach, Williams was a great experience for me. Medical school is hard, but what prepared me for it the most, even more than my organic chemistry lab, was the basketball program." That's the kind of letter I live for.

Aaron Dupuis was another bench player with a tremendous work ethic. When I recruited him, I said, "You have to worry about two things. You might be a step slow. And you're a local kid, so you'll be watched closely by everyone in town." Undaunted, he came in and worked his rear end off, and he improved vastly, although he never played much in games.

Aaron said, "I want to make the team better on Saturday night, so I'm going to work hard on Tuesday, Wednesday, and Thursday." And that's what he did. Every day he walked into the locker room and pulled on his shorts and shirt, knowing he was going to go out there for two hours to compete. He understood his role and knew his value to the team. He made our reserves a competitive group by the sheer force of his will. When Aaron wasn't there, it showed. Once he was hurt for about two weeks, and the intensity of our practices took a nosedive. I told the other players, "If we have to have Aaron on the court for you to be competitive, then we have a problem. Because he can't do it for you right now." I'm sure that it meant a lot to Aaron to have me say that in front of the entire team and coaching staff. He was one of the most respected players on our team, and his ex-teammates hold him in high regard to this day.

> *Passion and excitement come first. Work ethic will follow.*

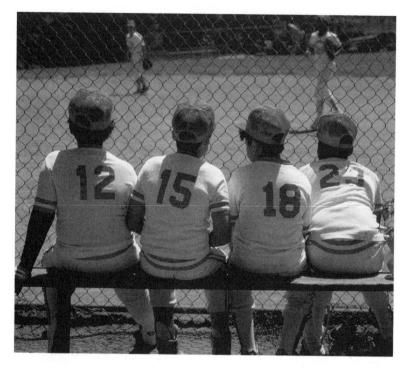

Many coaches are fixated on results. The basic mistake most make in regard to work ethic is not recognizing the contributions of nonstarters like Seth and Aaron in front of their teammates. In a basketball game, not every player plays; not every player is on the floor when it counts, when there are people in the stands, when there is noise in the gym, when there is an excitement he wants to be a part of. These players don't hear their names shouted by the fans; they won't see their achievements written up in the papers. But some of these kids make tremendous contributions to the team. So as the coach, *you* have to acknowledge these players, in a way that really means something to them. Take the time to stop practice and recognize their hard work in front of their teammates and coaches. It's the most important recognition they can get. Their teammates are their brothers, their fraternity. And if a player gets positive feedback from a group he really cares about, he will do almost anything for them.

■ ■ ■

WHEN I WAS IN HIGH SCHOOL, A BOY NAMED BOBBY GALVIN LIVED down the street from me. He was a couple of years younger than me, and when I started making a name for myself on the basketball team, he started gravitating toward me because he wanted to be a player, too. He figured that if *I* could succeed through hard work, anybody could. When I was hired as athletic director at Williams College in 2000, Bobby heard about it, and he dropped me a note. He congratulated me and recalled our time spent in the park together, working on our game. I was sad to learn that he had never had success in the sport and had given it up, but he wrote something really perceptive about that: "Harry, I didn't need to become a great basketball player. I just needed to be there, practicing. I learned that there is something innately valuable about working hard. At that time in my youth, it was important to have that discipline."

We must often remind parents and coaches that their kids are playing games, not performing brain surgery. But as Bobby said, there is a certain time in a young person's life when there is something extremely valuable about working hard in order to stretch and achieve some level of self-fulfillment. It has been my experience that kids who accomplish something they are proud of through hard work adopt work ethic as one of their core values. And a work ethic can carry a young person a good long way through life.

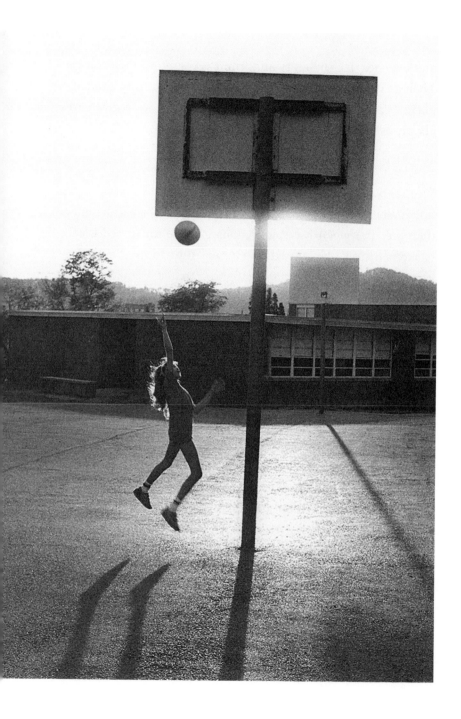

GOAL SETTING

If work ethic is the foundation for improvement in sports and in life, then goals are the building blocks. Hard work will bring some results, but it's not nearly as efficient as hard work coupled with a goal. To be productive, work must have a focus. A kid wouldn't have much of a chance of making ninety percent of his free throws if he just threw the basketball up in the air; she'd never be able to convert seventy percent of her field goal attempts if she kicked the ball in no particular direction; he'd never achieve an A in history if he checked off the multiple-choice answers without reading the questions. If you're not focused, any good result is accidental. The point is: You have to have a target to hit a target. You need a goal.

It's a shame how many kids with a good work ethic float through their athletic existence without any notion of what they want to achieve, much less how to get there. As a coach, my biggest challenge was working with players who didn't know how to set goals to improve their skills. Such kids need direction to get them really excited about a sport, and it's the job of coaches — ideally with support from parents — to inspire them with focus and purpose.

The ability to set good goals is not a gift received at birth but an acquired skill that has to be developed. Adults *must* teach kids how to set goals. The younger a child learns this lesson, the better off he or she will be. And here's where athletics proves important. Being involved in a sport provides kids with an ideal opportunity to develop their goal-setting skills. All the players I've known who learned to set smart goals in basketball, baseball, football, soccer, and other sports brought this skill to other parts of their lives. Goal setting is a life skill, and kids should understand its value.

■ ■ ■

FOR A GOAL TO BE GOOD, IT MUST BE BOTH MEASURABLE AND obtainable. Goals should make you stretch to achieve them, but they should also be realistic. There is no satisfaction in reaching a goal that isn't challenging, but not being able to reach a goal is discouraging. Setting good goals is a real art, which is why an adult — a coach, parent, or teacher — should be involved. I believe that parents should initiate the process. It's a good way for them to get involved in their kid's athletic experience, and keeping track of goals can help parents stay in touch with what their kid is really learning from teammates, coaches, practices, and games. To get started, all parents have to do is sit down with their child and say, "Are you excited about this season? Let's go over your goals. Then you can talk to your coach about them."

Most important, goals should be written down. When I was a boy, I went to a camp where a coach told us kids to write down our goals. I discovered that this was a great motivator for me. It's in my nature to need to know where I stand, and from then on I was always keeping track of my goals. Writing them down made them real. I posted them on my mirror or kept them in my notebook, where I could see them frequently. I also kept a free-throwing chart over my bed. Every day I took one hundred free throws at the park, and when I got back home I'd write down how many of those shots I had made that day.

Having seen how helpful this was to me, I tell kids at my camps, "If you want to be a player, keep a notebook to remind you of your goals and to show you if you have gotten any better than you were last month, last week, or the day before yesterday." I don't tell the kids that they must keep a notebook. Some of them might not want to be players, and it's not up to any coach or parent to legislate passions. But if kids are really excited a sport — or any other activity, for that matter — they really will

For a goal to be good, it must be both measurable and obtainable.

find it both helpful and fun to get a notebook and keep records of their workouts so they can see how quickly they are progressing toward their goals. They can also use the notebook as an inspirational scrapbook, pasting in it quotations, articles, photos — whatever has a positive impact on them. Of course, on their own, kids aren't likely to say, "Hey, I should keep a notebook." It's the job of parents and coaches to recommend it to them.

It was always my practice to ask new players on my team to make a list of four basketball goals, as well as four academic goals. I was amazed at how few of these bright kids wrote down sound, measurable, obtainable goals. Many would say, "I want to be a better shooter" or "I want to become a better

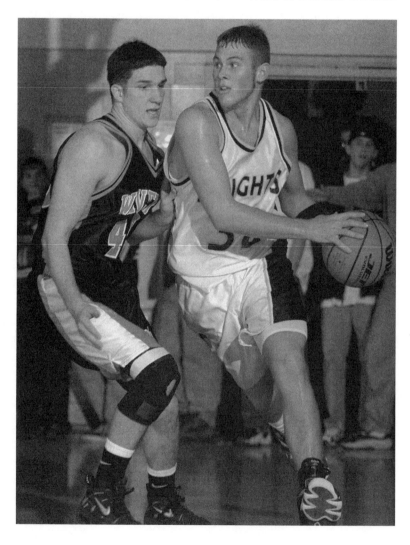

rebounder." I'd have to tell them that their goals were too fuzzy. How would we be able to tell at the end of the year if they had really improved? I'd encourage them to set goals that we could measure. For instance, a player might write, "My goal is to earn eighteen minutes of playing time per game, which is reasonable if I work hard. Playing eighteen minutes, I'd like to shoot forty percent from the floor, grab eight rebounds, and make seventy-five percent of my free throws." Those are great goals. After a few games, we would get together to reevaluate these goals. If the player was shooting fifty percent from the floor, we realized that forty percent was too easy a goal, and we'd set a new goal of, say, fifty-five percent. If he was shooting sixty percent from the foul line, we had to decide whether seventy-five percent was a realistic goal, and if so, we'd devise a workout plan for him to get there.

It's a tremendous boost for a player to have his coach and his parents know his goals and invest in them. Parents and coaches can't make those goals happen, but they can help the kid reach them. For example, if I knew players wanted to shoot better, I would encourage them to take one hundred extra shots after practice every day, and I would rebound for them. Grateful that I was investing my time to help them achieve a goal, they would work harder to do just that.

■ ■ ■

A GOAL SHOULD REFLECT YOUR VALUE SYSTEM. IF I WERE THE pastor of my church and my goal didn't mesh with what I do — perhaps I wanted to become rich enough to buy the most expensive house in town — then I would have to stop and reconsider. Are my goals leading me toward the type of person I want to be? A young basketball player who tells his parents or coach, "I want to average forty points a game," reveals that he values his individual achievements over his team's goals. He is being neither realistic nor unselfish enough to fit into the team-oriented game most coaches want to have. Individual players must have individual goals, but individual goals must support team goals.

Williams College had a heck of a men's soccer team in 2000, including sophomore Alex Blake, one of the best players in the country. Alex had set a goal of scoring two or three goals a game, which was not impossible considering his immense talent. But in one game when the team was winning by five goals, Coach Mike Russo took Alex out early. Alex had scored only once and was noticeably upset. That was a chance for Coach Russo to sit down with Alex and talk about the quality of his goal. He explained that when the games were close, he had no problem leaving in his star and would want him to try to score his two or three goals, and even more. But if the team was blowing out their opponent, Coach Russo wouldn't play his star for the entire game. He wanted to give bench players a chance to play and develop their skills. It all sank in, and Alex really started to understand that team goals must supercede individual goals — and that there is absolutely no feeling that surpasses what you experience

> *Team goals must supercede individual goals — and there is absolutely no feeling that surpasses what you experience when you achieve goals as a team.*

when you achieve goals as a team. When Alex broke Williams's career scoring record the next year, as a junior, he said sincerely, "The reason I broke the record is that I have the best teammates in the country. I simply converted the opportunities they provided me."

■　■　■

DURING THE FINAL YEARS OF MY TENURE AS HEAD MEN'S BASKET-ball coach at Williams, I was fortunate to have on my team a great player named Michael Nogelo. In 1995, when he was a freshman, I called Michael into my office and asked him to write down his primary goal. He wrote, "I am going to work hard and become an All-American." I said, "That's a good goal for you." It was a lofty goal, but for Michael it was in reach, and I told him that I would help him try to achieve it. Two days later, I walked into the gym and found him playing one-on-one with another player, and he was just goofing around and flinging the ball from all over the gym. Michael had a great work ethic and a good goal, but it was obvious that what was missing was a *plan* that would keep him focused enough to achieve his goal. So we came up with a directed plan in which he was never to take his practice time casually and he was to work hard to improve every aspect of his game in measurable ways. The plan didn't mean that Michael couldn't have fun; he simply needed to bring focus to his enjoyment of the game. After that, Michael bore down, and in 1998 he became not only an All-American but also National Player of the Year.

If you ask people if they have goals in life, most will answer yes. However, when you press them, you'll discover that even if they have realistic goals, few have concrete plans for reaching them. If I had a son and wanted to help him realize his goal of improving academically, I might tell him: "We're going to spend forty minutes studying together three nights a week, covering a different subject each time. And every weekend we're going to watch one television show that relates to a subject you're studying, and afterward we'll talk about it." Then we would have a viable plan for achieving better grades. In sports, too, adults need to help each child not only come up with suitable goals but also formulate smart, time-efficient plans for reaching them. A plan gives a young athlete the day-to-day commitment that is necessary to achieve a goal.

A reasonable goal in baseball may be to raise your batting average. That sounds simple enough; you want to get from batting average A to batting average B. But we tend to forget that there are a lot of small steps in between that make up the plan to reach B. It might be that you will first take fifty extra swings a day, then move to one hundred a day, and then move from hitting soft tosses to hitting against a pitching machine. You might spend more and more time learning to hit to the opposite field and to hit off-speed pitching. A basketball player wanting to improve his shooting may first go from shooting one hundred shots a day after practice to shooting two hundred; then he'll start shooting at a game pace so that he can get his shots off quickly. Each step of the plan that takes you from A to B is probably more difficult than you would have expected.

Once a player knows the proper technique for shooting a basketball — hip, elbow, and wrist in line; shoot the ball up toward the basket; follow through — there's no complexity to the process of becoming a better shooter. It's just a matter of repetition and shooting at game speed. It's really that simple. But if it were easy, every youth, high school, and college player would take five hundred extra shots a day, and every one of them would become good shoot-

ers. Along the way, players find out that *simple* doesn't mean *easy*. It takes hard work, perseverance, and determination to follow through on a plan. Often it's *not* easy. When I was a boy struggling through my daily workouts, my dad told me something that has stuck with me: When all is said and done, usually a lot more has been said than done. We've all heard people say they have a goal and a plan for reaching it, but once the hard

> *Going up a mountain is much harder than staying at the bottom, but when you get to the top, the view is so much better.*

work starts, the plan is often abandoned and the goal is forgotten. *Saying* you're going to reach a goal is simple; actually *doing* it is not. Recognizing this, parents and coaches must get involved in their kids' goal-setting. By helping kids follow through on their plans, you'll show them that goal-setting is a powerful tool for developing skills and building pride.

In 1983 I had a player named Tim Walsh. He was about 5'9" and probably didn't weigh 150 pounds, but he was dedicated and mentally tough. He was the kind of kid who would say, "Coach, I'm going to take five hundred shots a day," and then actually do it. Some kids will make that kind of promise and then never step into the gym. But Tim knew that his success depended on work, so he spent time every day after practice shooting a basketball, and he became an outstanding shooter. Moreover, he practiced dribbling for so many hours that you honestly couldn't tell if he was right- or left-handed. Tim worked incredibly hard to reach a high level of play. If it were easier than that, more people would do it. The people who are willing to work hard and make sacrifices while pursuing a difficult goal are the same people who will reach it. As I have told my players and campers for many years: Going up a mountain is much harder than staying at the bottom, but when you get to the top, the view is so much better.

Athletes are sometimes reluctant to set goals because they fear they can't reach them. They worry that if they set a goal and come up short, it will reflect badly on them as players. But

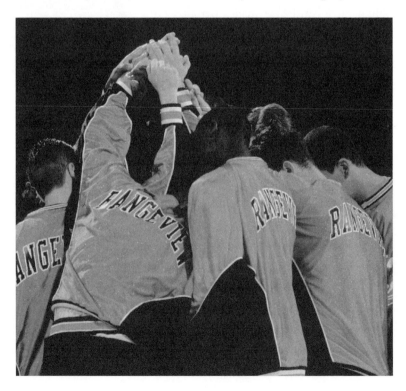

what young athletes don't understand — and parents and coaches are often as naïve — is that there is no reason why a goal can't be adjusted. Say a player told me he wanted to average eighteen points and nine rebounds a game, and I told him that was a reachable goal. But after a few games, we saw that while his rebound goal had been realistic, our style of play as a team prevented him from averaging more than ten points a game. Rather than saying his original goal for points was foolish or that he wasn't performing as he should, we would come up with a new goal based on my offensive philosophy and, of course, his playing time and role when he was on the floor. There is no disgrace in changing a goal. There are so many factors that affect an athlete's performance, and many of them are beyond his control.

> *When a goal disappears, it must be replaced by a new one.*

One of the best athletes I ever had at Williams was a 6'5" kid named John Botti. He injured his knee in a game against UMass-Dartmouth in the NCAA tournament in March 1995, tearing both ligaments and cartilage. After he had surgery, I told John that we needed a plan to get him back in the shortest period of time possible without damaging the knee. Our goal was for him to be ready to play on November 1, when our new year began. John was amazing. He rode twenty to thirty miles on a stationary bike every day. He put on a rubber harness and dragged one of the coaches around the gym, walking backward because it was pain free, and gradually increasing the number of circuits he made. I had him do his rehabilitation work in view of the other players during practice; it inspired them to see what he was going through in order to play. In addition, we put together a shooting progression for him, having him make the transition from taking 50 to 100 to 250 shots within twenty-five minutes, a real fitness workout. He did this day after day after day.

John was coming along well, but in October he hit a snag, developing tendonitis. So we changed our goal to January 9, our first game after winter break. Rather than shut down after this disappointment, John said that he would stick to his routine, except that he wouldn't shoot for two weeks, to give himself time to heal. On January 9, he made his comeback, playing six minutes in three two-minute spurts. By February he was starting again. And one year to the day after he was injured, again in the NCAA tournament, again against UMass-Dartmouth, he made a great defensive steal, in the exact spot on the floor where he had been injured. He laid the ball in, was fouled, and made the free throw, and we won the game to qualify for the Sweet Sixteen.

You have to have a target to hit a target.

I don't think John would have gotten so far without knowing how to set goals and measure his improvement. We kept track of everything, even the number of times he pulled someone around the gym. His rehabilitation was painful and difficult, and when it made sense to adjust his goals, he did, with guidance from myself, the director of sports medicine, and a lot of other people who were invested in his goals. But despite setbacks and frustration, John didn't give up. His goal at the beginning of the season might have been to become an All-New England player, but after the injury, it was just being able to play again. Life is funny that way; it changes when you least expect it and requires constant adjustments. John took that lesson to heart. As much as he suffered, I believe that John really values the experience of having reached a truly challenging, difficult goal.

■ ■ ■

PLAYERS CAN ACCELERATE THEIR IMPROVEMENT BY WRITING down their goals and devising a plan for reaching them. However, once players reach their goals, parents and coaches can't allow them to become complacent. The fundamental rule of goal setting is this: When a goal disappears, it must be replaced by a new one.

Teach kids not to be satisfied with their skill levels but to try to constantly improve, to consider themselves always to be a work in progress. They will soon learn that they can control their own destiny by setting goals, having a plan, and going to work.

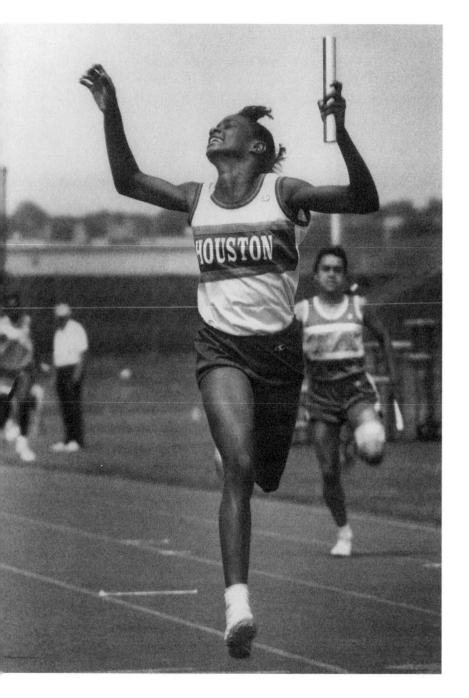

SUCCESS

There is a closed box on my desk with a sign on top that reads, "The Secret of Success." When someone opens the box, they find the answer: "Hard Work."

I wholeheartedly believe that the secret of success is hard work, but after seventeen years of coaching college players and grade-school campers, I've come to realize that for the majority of young athletes and their parents, and even for some coaches, the definition of success itself is a secret. Few parents can define for their children and themselves what the hard work is going to lead to, and few can recognize when their youngsters experience success in a sport. For some kids, it's playing just a few minutes or a few innings every game; for others, it's being selected for the all-star team. For hard-working Seth Mehr, success was earning ten minutes of playing time on a Williams team that qualified for the NCAA tournament, but for an All-American-caliber player like Michael Nogelo, that wouldn't have been success at all. Success is different for every young athlete, and it should be defined by the goals individual players set with their coaches.

░ ░ ░

WHEN YOUNG ATHLETES REACH GOALS, SOMETIMES THEY AREN'T motivated to reach any further. They wrongly assume that the goal marks the finish line. What they don't see is that their success is in only one specific area of one specific sport. While coaches and parents should praise kids for having been successful, they also should teach them that success is never a final result. If kids hope to experience *overall* success, they must keep improving and striving to reach their potential.

As I always tell young athletes, you will never have success unless you stretch yourself. If you're always in your "comfort zone," you're not achieving your full potential. Success is a matter of personal accountability; only you know whether you're capable of stretching yourself even more and becoming better at what you do. If you can say, "I know I can do better," yet choose to stay in your comfort zone, then you cannot claim to be having success, even though you may appear to be to some people.

░ ░ ░

ADULTS MUST REALIZE THAT, FOR YOUNG ATHLETES, SUCCESS IS experiencing a pattern of growth that helps them understand who they are in relation to their sports, coaches, and teammates; what their values are; and how they can inject those values into their conduct as athletes, family members, and community members. There's so much passion and intensity inside young girls and boys; by giving them an arena in which they can strive for success, sports facilitates the thrill of self-discovery. What is needed from these young athletes for this to happen? A continuous good effort. One might even say that a continuous good effort is the definition of success, because it teaches us so much about ourselves and how we want to live.

These concepts may be too heady to be comprehended by most young athletes, particularly those not yet in college. They'd rather think of success in the most simplistic terms. If you ask even the smartest young boys and girls what success is, most will exclaim, "Being rich and famous!" Wrong! When fame becomes the goal, then the positive journey, that continuous good effort that defines real

Success is never a final result.

success, stalls. If young players start mimicking famous prima donna athletes, both in showy style of play and cocky attitude, and it's clear that appearance has become more of a concern than playing the game correctly, then coaches and parents have the difficult job of getting them to refocus.

Let me make it clear: Success and fame are very different. But the media bombards our kids with glorified, romanticized stories of the rich and famous. Is it any wonder that they begin to believe that there is nothing more glamorous than celebrity status or more important than fame? We as coaches and parents get to spend just a few brief hours with our kids every day. In that time, we have to remind them of the difference between success and fame.

There are plenty of people who are *famous* but not *successful.* They've achieved fame but not good lives. It's easy to think of numerous famous athletes, television and movie stars, pop singers, and others in the public eye who have really messed up their lives. Look at Dennis Rodman, the former NBA star with the questionable attitude that resulted in a premature end to his career. A great rebounder with an unbelievable nose for the ball, Rodman was a wonderful player, but he achieved most of his fame by blatantly exploiting the outrageous way he looked and behaved. After a while the novelty wore off, he lost his NBA showcase, and every report we heard about his life was negative. He is famous, yes, but is he successful? Not in a broad sense. Those people who don't distinguish between fame and success might wish they could trade their lives for his. But I'm sure that if they examined Rodman's life under a microscope and discovered the turmoil, most would reconsider.

Of course, being famous doesn't mean that you can't also be successful. There are many professional athletes who do their jobs quietly and competently and live very successful personal lives. They know and are comfortable with who they are, and they have no need to run around telling everyone how great they are. In fact, some use their fame as a means for doing good. They contribute time and money to charities, do positive work in their communities, or just help friends and family who are in need. Take Bobby Jones as an example. Bobby was a star forward at the University of North Carolina and went on to have a great professional career in the short-lived ABA and then in the NBA, where he played several years with Julius Erving on the Philadelphia 76ers. He was a super player who achieved great

> *There are plenty of people who are famous but not successful.*

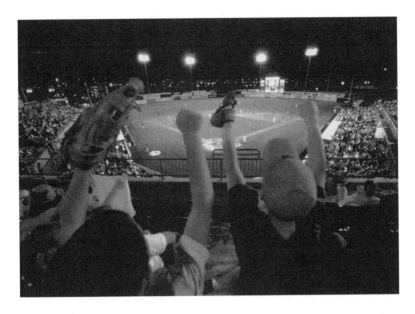

fame and made a lot of money, yet he remained true to his values. And he remained loyal to his friends, among whom was a former teammate from college, Brad Hoffman. In my first year with Athletes-in-Action, Brad was our point guard. Just before I joined the team, Brad's wife Becky gave birth to premature twins. They each weighed just a little over a pound and required much medical attention. The medical bills were immense. We all want appropriate credit for our good deeds, but Bobby Jones helped Brad and Becky pretty much anonymously. He very quietly paid a lot of bills and also set up a charity basketball game. I was very touched and impressed by his actions.

I had the chance to play against Bobby in later years, and I didn't have to be around him long to recognize that he was a very nice, clearly successful man. In character he was far removed from the egocentric athletes that we see so much of on television. Could Bobby have been like them? Absolutely. For example, he could have handled his assistance to Brad and Becky differently, alerting the media to let everyone know about his contribution. Nobody would have said a thing if he had; it fits the norm of how most professional athletes act. But he chose not to, and to me *that* spoke of success.

■ ■ ■

YOU CAN HAVE SUCCESS WITHOUT FAME AND FAME WITHOUT success. You can also have success and fame simultaneously. But they are always separate entities. Success, unlike fame, is a function of a high-quality life. That's important. You can have a very high-quality life without achieving fame. You can have fame but not necessarily a high-quality life.

Should fame ever be a goal? I don't think so. That's my value system. I want my plan for reaching a goal to be quality-oriented, not bogged down in a gray area that leaves me in danger of compromising my ethics. As I move toward my goal, I ask myself, "Is it worth it? Is this the right thing to do?" If fame were my goal, I fear I would have a different dynamic. Wanting to be famous leads us to actions different from those we would undertake if we wanted to be successful. For instance, if a kid decides he will work hard to become a famous athlete rather than to become a good team player, he will mostly likely play very selfishly. Fame has its merits for those who enjoy the public eye. But I believe that fame is much healthier as a by-product of success than as a goal.

Some people can achieve both success and fame, and that's terrific. But it is hard to do both. Fame brings with it a lot of demands and problems that tend to break down success. Being rich and famous doesn't equate with being happy. On the other hand, we all know people who don't have much money but live rich lives. They understand who they are, they operate within their sound value systems, and they are passing these values on to their kids. They find their lives to be challenging, fulfilling, and enjoyable, and that makes them content.

Contentment is not a characteristic of fame and money but of success, which means it's part of an ongoing process to improve skills and reach goals. If an athlete's goal is to achieve great fame and wealth, he probably will never be content. When will the wealth be enough? What happens when he can no longer play and the fame dies down?

I tell young athletes that there will come a time when they can no longer play the game. Even if they buck the odds and rise to stardom, in their hometown or across the nation, at some point they will enter a stage in their lives when they'll no longer see their name in the sports pages. Some athletes don't know how to handle this. Their entire model of success is built around sports, with dreams of winning championships, being famous, and becoming a highly paid professional athlete. I remind these players that they can draw from the sound principles they learned during their sports experiences. They can set new goals,

> *Success is a function of a high-quality life.*

make new plans, and always reach for the greater good in themselves. If they can do this — if we can teach these young kids how to get started on an ethical journey toward success — and they make that big, continuous effort to stay the course, they will have full, productive, joyful lives. There is no better goal.

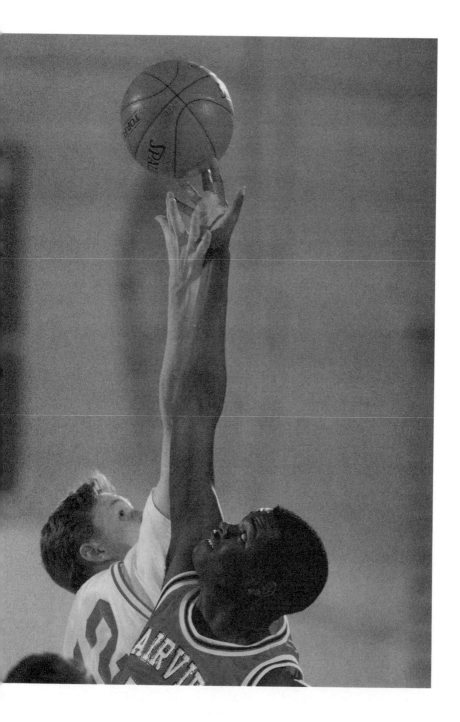

EXCELLENCE

I was very young when I developed a passion for sports, so there's no telling how many valuable lessons I learned on basketball courts and ball fields that I apply to other areas of my life. Likewise, I have learned much outside of sports that has proven essential to me in the athletic arena. For example, I began to reflect on the theme of excellence — which became a focal point of my playing, teaching, and living — after a quick visit to, of all places, a disheveled little radio station in Tulsa, Oklahoma, back in 1975.

After I graduated from college, I began a seven-year stint with the amateur basketball team Athletes in Action. We had a grueling schedule, playing the top college and amateur teams in the United States every day of the week. A game against the University of Tulsa allowed this easterner to visit Oklahoma for the first time. However, before I got to see Tulsa or the surrounding oil fields, a few of us were dispatched to a small radio station to plug the upcoming game.

I had never been inside a radio station and was curious to see this one. My excitement quickly gave way to disappointment. During our brief tour of the premises, I observed numerous boxes of clutter piled along the walls and recording tape that had unwound from the spool and ran from a table down to the floor. Anybody who walked into that station would have had the same negative reaction I did, which was, "My, there's a lot of junk around here!" I naïvely asked the guy taking us through the station what all that stuff was for — I assumed that it was out because it was used every day. However, our guide shrugged and said words I'd never forget, "Oh, that's just some old junk. We're just a small station and don't have a full staff to keep everything in order. We don't worry about it."

I remember thinking that the people who worked at the radio station were clearly underselling themselves. "We're just this" is a dangerous phrase. It's like a young athlete saying there's no point in working to improve because "I'm just small" or "I'm just slow." At that precise moment in the radio station, it dawned on me that far too many people will settle for mediocrity when, with a little effort, they could have excellence instead. And that's unfortunate, because there already is too much mediocrity in the world. We don't need more, do we? No. We need more excellence.

I don't care how understaffed that radio station was; the employees should have had enough pride in themselves and their work to have put that junk in boxes, taped them up, and labeled them. A little work and a minimum effort each day to keep things tidy and orderly was all that was needed to lift that station out of the depths of mediocrity. As modest as that sounds, it would have been enough, because excellence — as I came to understand it — isn't really about huge successes, fame, or wealth. You don't need to be a millionaire, a scholarship-level athlete, a CEO, or a Division I coach to experience excellence. It's there for all people who want to do the right things in their lives. If they had shown the initiative to forego the status quo, those underpaid employees in that small, obscure radio station could have had excellence. In making improvements, they would have set an obtainable goal, come up with a plan, and incorporated work ethic. Add a dose of pride in what they were doing and what they would accomplish, and they would have exhibited several of the key elements that comprise excellence.

Excellence is one of those things that you recognize when you see it but is hard to define. What is excellence? I think it's a way to look at the world, a way to do things, a way to operate our lives on a daily basis. It is reflected in the way we handle the day-to-day pieces of our lives, giving order and organization to them. A business executive may impress everyone with his creative ideas, but if anyone should get a look at his company's day-to-day operations — the financial records, the production processes, the way his employees interact — they might discover that everything is in disarray. That's not excellence. I always took pride in how structured my basketball practices at Williams were. I believe that if other coaches watched a few of my practices, they could have told me exactly what my coaching philosophy was. If they couldn't break down everything I was teaching offensively and defensively after seeing two or three practices, then I wasn't doing as well as I thought, and I certainly wasn't achieving excellence.

> *Excellence is more a state of mind than a state of circumstance.*

Practice is where excellence is most evident in sports. It's highly unlikely that a team will play an excellent game if its practices are slipshod. In fact, I haven't seen any excellent sports organization that didn't have a healthy perspective on preparation for games. Significantly, it is at practices that young players who take pride in their own abilities make the gigantic leap to feeling pride in the team. This happens when they run through practices that are well-planned, function smoothly, and show results. A day or two later, they feel even more pride in the team when the game plan is executed properly against a rival team. When a team is pursuing excellence, you will find that players are more than willing to continue to make sacrifices to benefit the group.

There is surely excellence on a team in which the players feel accountable to each other. That was the dynamic on the best basketball teams I coached at Williams. Those fifteen kids from different places and different backgrounds bonded with each other; you could see it during huddles, when they often clasped hands or put their arms around each other's shoul-

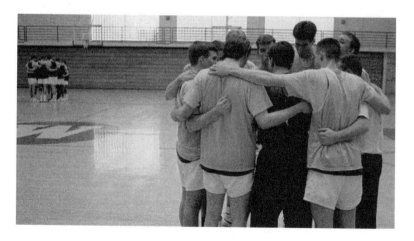

ders. Michael Nogelo, the All-American player who led one of those teams, felt responsible both on and off the court to his teammates who rarely played. Feeling appreciated by the National Player of the Year, those players would do anything for him and made sure never to do anything to embarrass him. As teammates, they were equals.

As a team, we spent hours and hours trying to do things the right way. We strove for excellence in both practices and games, and whether we won or lost, those young men lined up and shook hands with our opponents afterward. They knew that excellence is reflected in how you conduct yourself throughout your athletic experience, not just in how many games you win. In fact, you can exhibit excellence and still lose the game. For example, in my third year as head men's basketball coach at Williams, we beat a less-talented Brandeis team by about fifteen points, but I couldn't sleep all night because we didn't rebound or properly execute anything in our game plan. A few days later, we lost by seven points to Springfield, but since we played a great game against a team that was ranked fifth in Division II, I went home and slept like a baby. Sometimes you play an excellent game but the other team is just better.

> *Excellence is reflected in how you conduct yourself throughout your athletic experience, not just in how many games you win.*

For me, excellence implies an extended period of time, rather than one moment, one game, one season. Excellence is crafted through vision, planning, work, and determination; it is never an accident. You may have a good team for a year or two, but to have an excellent program you must have good teams for several years. Your kid may make a fantastic play in one game, but to be an excellent player he must be well-versed in the fundamentals, conduct himself with good humor and grace, and constantly strive to improve — every day, every practice, every game, every season.

But how are players to know that the work that goes into improving is as valuable as their performance if we, as adults, are interested only in the score of the game? If you want your child to know that practices are just as important as games, talk to him about them. Ask him, "How was practice today? What did the team work on? What did you learn?" Get out and practice with your kid at home. Set up games and drills; let your kid practice against you, or simply keep score or time or set the ball back up on the tee for him. By becoming involved in your kid's pursuit of excellence, you'll encourage both his skills and his enthusiasm.

■ ■ ■

WE LOOK FOR EXCELLENCE FROM THE OUTSIDE, BUT IT BEGINS ON the inside. It is more a state of mind than a state of circumstance. It is about how we appear to ourselves, who we think we really are. Kids don't know their own potential. They don't realize that they can get up in the morning and look in the mirror and be excited about the day ahead. They have no idea how much excellence they have in them or how much they can give if it is demanded of them. It's frustrating to watch them stagnate. They don't know how much they can push themselves — and that's usually much more than they think they can. As a parent, you are lucky if your child has a gifted coach or teacher who can help him understand excellence, and help him extract it. But it's your job, too.

John Wooden, a remarkable motivator who coached the UCLA men's basketball team to ten national championships, didn't like the common expression, "He gives 110 percent." So many coaches use that phrase, but you can't really sell it to a kid, because it's phony. Wooden said he was happy to get ninety percent from players, because most kids give only sixty percent on their own. Striving to reach your potential is about getting as close to one hundred percent as you can. Some kids do get close, but since perfection is impossible, their work is never done.

Parents and coaches must emphasize to their kids that excellence is about the small things. It's about giving order to what you do or are trying to accomplish. It is also about understanding your role on your team, in your classroom, in your business, or even in your family. When you tell your kid "Be yourself," you're asking her to excel at being who she is, to put into order the day-to-day details that are important to her. For myself, I want to be an excellent Harry, not an excellent Joe or an excellent Sarah. There already is a Joe and a Sarah, and it's their job to be who they are. My job is to be excellent in my own particular slot in life.

Achieving excellence is not easy, and for some, it can be quite difficult. But with encouragement and guidance, all kids can begin the journey toward excellence. No matter what challenges they face, a simple first step toward improvement will set them on the right path. Athletics provides an arena in which to begin that journey. That's the beauty of sports: It's one gigantic opportunity for self-improvement.

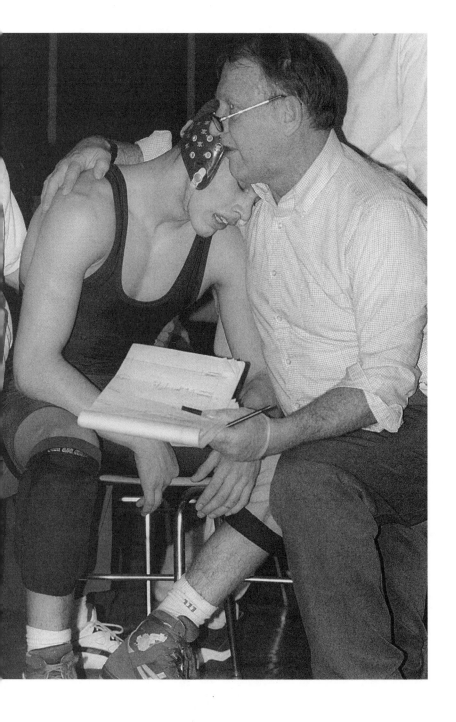

WINNING & LOSING

As a boy I took countless car rides with my father. He made his living as a stockbroker, but he coached baseball and basketball and played semipro ball, so we were always driving to games. On those memorable trips, he spoke passionately and eloquently about the two sports he loved most. He told me, "Harry, there is nothing like waking up on the day of a basketball game or going to the ballpark on a beautiful summer night." He pointed out that "it should be a blast" for anyone to play any sport, whatever the outcome. Significantly, he didn't think it was necessary to discuss winning or losing, other than to tell me to handle either result in a dignified manner. Instead he talked about the thrill of playing the game, the importance of being a good teammate, and the satisfaction of improving through work.

Today, it's rare that a young athlete has a parent or coach who can convey to him that winning and losing are not what is most important about the game. I was fortunate in that I was given wise counsel by one of each. My Little League coach, John Bardong, had views similar to those of my father. Coach Bardong, as I still call him, made my experience positive because he understood that baseball is primarily a great game for kids to learn and have fun playing. He taught me that both wins and losses have only temporary impact and importance, and that you shouldn't get hung up on the outcome of any one game because there is always another game ahead and another one after that. Under Coach Bardong's watchful eye, my team-mates and I never thought, "Oh, my gosh, we *have* to win this game!" Without that worry, we were able to play loose and have fun, and — it wasn't just coincidence — we had an out-standing win-loss record.

I went on to junior high and played on teams that didn't win very often. That I survived through that time with my enthusiasm for sports intact was due in large part to what I

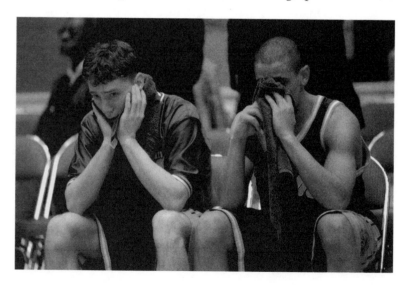

had learned from my father and Coach Bardong. I drew from those sound lessons and told myself, "Okay, I'm just going to work hard this season to improve my skills. Next season will be better." As the losses mounted, it was my love of the game that kept me going. I don't know what percentage of kids give up on a sport because they can't handle losing; from my experience, it seems like a significant number. But what my father and Coach Bardong taught me at a very young age enabled me to have a healthy perspective on winning and losing, which has helped me as a player in youth, college, and professional sports and then as a coach.

■ ■ ■

IN SEVENTEEN YEARS OF COACHING AT WILLIAMS, MY TEAMS WON seventy-five percent of our games, in large part because they had developed a healthy attitude toward winning and losing. I had good players who understood that winning isn't a ticket to paradise and losing isn't death. After some tough losses, I joked, "It hurts me, it hurts you, but it'll be at least two days before they get word of our loss in China. Of course they'll be disappointed, but at least we'll have a few days before they get the bad news." And whether we won or lost it was, "Hey, guys, you have class tomorrow." It was important to me that they kept things in perspective.

I don't deny that as a college coach I preferred winning over losing. Winning certainly made my job easier. What I wanted my players to understand—and what all coaches, parents, and kids should understand—is that there can be as much worth in losing as there is in winning and as many negatives in winning as in losing. We adults may contend, "Kids will learn lessons no matter what transpires," but unless those same kids actually buy into our atypical (for this day and age) view on winning and losing, it's unlikely that they will know how to handle either properly. If we really want kids to understand that the game itself is more important than who won or lost, the first question out of our mouths when a young child walks in through the door after a game can't be "Did you win?" In fact, it must not be even the second, third, or fourth question we ask.

■ ■ ■

VERY YOUNG BOYS AND GIRLS SHOULD PLAY GAMES JUST FOR FUN; in some leagues, they don't even keep track of the score, and that's not a bad idea. However, as young athletes mature and begin to understand the real values of the game, the scoreboard can become a good measure of progress. One of the real joys of competing is finding out how well you can perform against other teams. Winning as a team then can become a good goal.

Conscientious parents know that they shouldn't put too much pressure on their kids to win and that they should try to teach their kids to accept a loss with grace. However, as a parent, coach, or player, your attitude should never be that it's okay to lose. Trying to accomplish something as a team is a significant undertaking, and after days of practice and preparation, that includes making a concerted effort — competing as hard as you can — to achieve a victory. If you fail, it's natural to feel disappointed. A coach, parent, or player who is completely demoralized by a loss doesn't have a healthy perspective on the game; on the other hand, someone who simply laughs off a loss devalues what the team is doing.

Unfortunately, many people think that the scoreboard is the only valid measure of a game and have a terribly negative reaction to losing. It's true that the scoreboard can seem like a huge monster, sitting up high and blaring the news of your loss to all the world. However, there are hundreds of ways to measure the success of a game. For instance, the team may lose the game, but one player may pull down seventeen rebounds when his goal was only ten, or make five solo tackles when the goal was just two. Even after defeats, such efforts must be acknowledged.

■ ■ ■

JUST BECAUSE A TEAM PUT MORE POINTS ON THE SCOREBOARD than their opponent doesn't mean that they won well. There are different types of winning, and they reflect on the character of the coaches and players. There are wrong ways to win. Obviously a coach and his players shouldn't try to win by cheating, bending the rules, or doing anything else unethical. A coach with integrity does not play kids who are over the age limit, bring in "ringers," or give less talented kids less playing time than the league prescribes. He doesn't have his kids fake injuries for whatever reason or allow them to try to injure the star players of the opposing team. And he doesn't devise sneaky "trick" plays that border on being illegal or not inform game officials when an officiating mistake has been made because it benefits his team. Winning is not so important that a coach should do any of these things, or worse.

> *It is your response to winning and losing that makes you a winner or a loser.*

The attitude of the players on the winning team has a lot to do with the quality of the win. Poor sportsmanship — grandstanding, taunting, or any other display of disrespect for opponents, fans, or officials — during and after games takes away from victories and can tarnish an otherwise stellar performance. The only thing worse than a poor loser is a poor winner. And believe me, there are plenty of them out there.

Another less-than-glorious way to win is to have played with a disappointing output of focus and effort. That's when you win with a small "w." The losses that most upset me were those in which I felt the team's effort just wasn't there. Again, I think back to when my Williams team edged a weak Brandeis basketball team and then lost a close game to a highly ranked Springfield squad. When we beat Brandeis, we succeeded in the world's eyes, but we failed in mine because of our poor effort. When we lost to Springfield, we failed in everyone else's eyes but shone in mine because we played hard against a more athletic, more skilled team. I also remember a triple-overtime game that ended when the other team picked up a loose ball and hit a 25-foot desperation shot at the buzzer. We lost on the scoreboard, but my kids couldn't possibly have given any more of themselves, and I was proud of our winning effort.

■ ■ ■

A GAME IS A TEST OF HOW WELL THE TEAM HAS PREPARED IN PRACtice. However, at the end of the "test," if the number on your side of the scoreboard turns out to be less than the number on the opponent's side, that doesn't mean that the team failed the exam. The "test" evaluates more than the final score. It has to, because sooner or later you are going to come up against a team that is simply better than you are. When that's the case, if we continue to insist that the only way to pass the "test" is to win, then we're doomed to failure. Parents, coaches, and players have to find ways other than the score to measure the success of a team. For example, as a coach I might give my basketball team a passing grade if we outhustled the other team, made only a few turnovers, accumulated a certain number of offensive rebounds, or reached any number of other goals we'd set. As a parent, you might consider your daughter's softball game a successful one if she kept her temper all

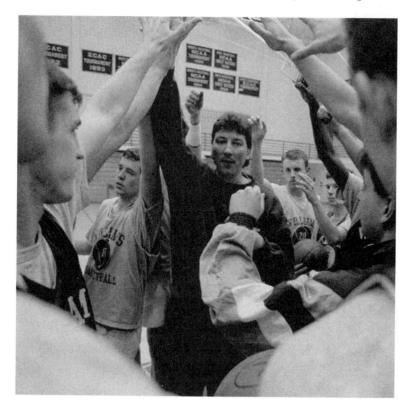

the way through, she laid down a beautiful bunt when asked to, and twice the team, with runners from the opposing team on first and third, defended against the steal — something they'd been having trouble with.

In our win-enamored society, we lose all sense of perspective by looking only at the final score. If a team wins by a score of 83–82, they might recap the game by saying how well they had executed the game plan. But if they didn't make that last basket and they lost 82–81, they're more likely to say that they didn't box out, they didn't defend, they had a total breakdown in execution for the entire game. We are so caught up in winning and losing that when it comes down to the last second, we often base our evaluation of a team's performance for the full game on whether the last-second shot bounces in or out. Foolish, right? Yes, because the team's performance is essentially the same.

> *The only thing worse than a poor loser is a poor winner.*

As a society that is incredibly enthusiastic about sports, we must come to grips with our attitude toward winning and losing, because we're saddling kids with a huge responsibility — to win at all costs — when instead they should be having fun and learning life skills.

Kids see that in our culture losing is held in great disregard. Even second-place teams are shunned and forgotten. At the highest levels of sports, so much money is at stake that losing is unacceptable. Winning championships in college and the pros means millions of dollars in revenues. This sort of system might make it seem worth trying anything — even cheating — to win. We have to take a determined and vocal stand against this attitude, because it's out of control. This is a revolution that must trickle *up*, from the ten-year-olds who, with the help of adults, can make the distinction between youth sports and high-level college and professional sports, where winning is strictly business. Because with the lunacy at the top, it isn't going to trickle *down*.

■ ■ ■

MANY YOUTH, HIGH SCHOOL, AND COLLEGE COACHES TRY TO motivate their players by quoting Vince Lombardi, who said, "Winning isn't everything. It's the only thing." With this philosophy, Lombardi built an NFL dynasty in the 1960s with the Green Bay Packers. But what many coaches fail to take into account is that Lombardi was trying to motivate extraordinarily skilled, highly paid professionals. You simply can't motivate young athletes — whether they're eight or eighteen — in the same way. Sure, Lombardi's famous words can get a player all fired up. But what happens when the team loses? Will the young player have enough perspective on winning to know that losing is not the end of the world?

I believe that many people misinterpret Lombardi. If winning on the scoreboard really is the only thing, then the implication is that players should do whatever it takes to beat their opponents — even stray outside the rules. That's something Lombardi never would have condoned. Lombardi was a master motivator and character-builder, and I prefer to believe that he was thinking of winning both on and off the scoreboard. After all, when he brought his players together for inspirational talks, he spoke to them in metaphors about life — not football.

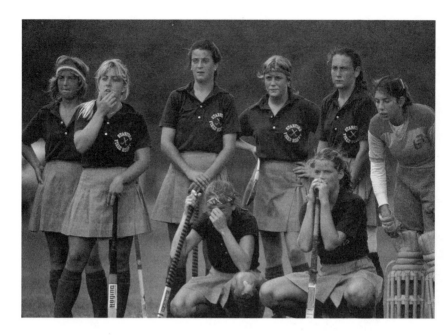

Winning on the scoreboard is quite different from winning off the scoreboard, that is, improving yourself by playing the game. Winning on the scoreboard cements and builds a young player's confidence in himself and his team. It proves, as good coaches insist, that a big victory can be a by-product of doing a lot of little things right. It also confirms that a coach's practices and game plans have merit. However, when coaches or parents overemphasize winning, they're setting their kids up for failure—in sports, losing is unavoidable. Better results come from telling kids that great teams play hard and with intensity, yet relaxed and loose. I love to see kids play with intensity, but when kids are told that losing is unacceptable, that intensity often becomes tension. When young players are not afraid to lose, they are more apt to play well, and they'll enjoy themselves more.

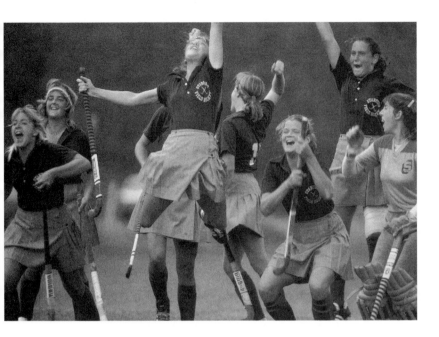

The biggest question about winning versus losing is: Do you control it, or does it control you? When young people see adults who are equally controlled after wins and losses, the impact on them is strong. And when players don't get too high after winning or too low after losing, they are able to operate in a zone that is comfortable and productive.

■ ■ ■

I ASK KIDS AT MY CAMPS, "WHAT'S GOOD ABOUT LOSING?" THEY often can't think of a thing. So I'll tell them that they have to experience losing in order to know why they want to win. If you could only win or tie, the game would have a completely different dynamic, and winning wouldn't have much value. And there are lessons to be learned from losing. In fact, I'd say that we learn more about ourselves after our losses than after our wins.

Character is revealed most after a loss. Losing exposes you, bringing up every vile thing that's in you. People are going to know who you are after a tough loss. For instance, if you're a coach who rants and raves against the officials at a post-game press conference, that's going to tell people an awful lot about how you view winning and losing.

Losing can crush egos. It diminishes how we feel about ourselves more than it should, just as winning gives us a bigger boost than it should. I'm as guilty as anyone else of letting winning give me an inflated ego. For instance, when my Williams team was in the middle of a fifty-one-game win streak at home, I felt as though we were invincible in our gym. I thought I could throw our sneakers out on the court and we'd win. Then we were upset by Trinity College, and I was dropped back down to earth. It's amazing how dramatically that one loss after fifty-one wins attacked how we felt about ourselves as a team.

But one of the great things about sports is that after you lose, most of the time you get to play again soon. After our loss to Trinity, I told my players, "You have two choices on how to react to this loss: You either wallow in it or bounce. There is no middle ground." The next game we went out and played one of the best halves of basketball I've ever seen a team play at any level. We were up 51–26 at the half against Amherst College, a big rival that had beaten us the first time we played them. I was so proud of my players. Of course, like any coach, part of me wanted to look back and think, "Well, if we'd played like that against Trinity, we would have annihilated them, too." But that's not the lesson that needs to be learned! So instead I congratulated my players, saying, "Instead of letting our loss to

Trinity demoralize you, guys, you bounced back and came out stronger. You should be proud of yourselves."

Some of my favorite moments as a player and as a coach have been after losses. Those are real teaching and learning moments. You never have your kids' attention as much as when you lose. When the team is winning, kids think you're crying wolf if you tell them that they must work hard to improve. But when you lose, you have their undivided attention, and they are willing to change. Some of the biggest improvements you can make as a player or coach is when the team is going through a tough time. In 1998, for example, my team lost our final regular season game against Hamilton College. It cost us the top seed in the northeast regional bracket of the NCAA tournament. However, we ended up facing Hamilton again in the tournament. Our loss to them a week before proved beneficial, because when we practiced for the rematch I had every ounce of my kids' attention. They were so focused that we easily won the second game, 91–69.

You never have your kids' attention as much as when you lose. Those are real teaching and learning moments.

If you can help kids look at losing as an opportunity to improve, you can help them make dramatic strides. Any kind of setback — athletic, professional, financial, or otherwise — can be difficult to overcome. But losses, failures, and adversity create new opportunities. When my wife Connie graduated from college, she was really intent on becoming a buyer for Gimbel's, the large department store chain. But she didn't get that job of her dreams, and she ended up going in a totally different direction, working in college administration. Would she have been happy with the Gimbel's job? Maybe. But she sure loves what she's doing now. A setback like that simply allows you an opportunity that you weren't expecting. There's an old saying that goes, "When one door closes, another one opens," and in my experience, that's been true. Some people experience truly devastating setbacks, and they can be difficult to overcome. But what sports teaches is that we can't let all of life's little setbacks stop our progress and steal our focus. In every setback there is something to learn and an opportunity to explore.

■　■　■

KIDS OFTEN REACT VERY EMOTIONALLY TO LOSING AND CAN have a hard time accepting it. For instance, my good friend's ten-year-old son just hates to lose. Every time he loses, he melts down. It's great that he competes so hard to win, but it's hard to stand by and watch him lose control of his emotions. Unfortunately, you can't put an on–off switch on a kid like that and just flip it, saying, "Don't feel like that!" It's okay if a kid cries when he loses — it shows that he has passion for the game and cares about the outcome — but it's not okay for a kid to throw a tantrum. As a coach or parent, it's your responsibility to teach him to deal with the emotional ups and downs of sports.

Most kids will wake up the day after a bad loss and it's as though it never happened. But at the heartbreaking moment, it's hard for a parent to watch. Pay attention, parents, because *that* difficult moment is the teaching moment, not the next day when

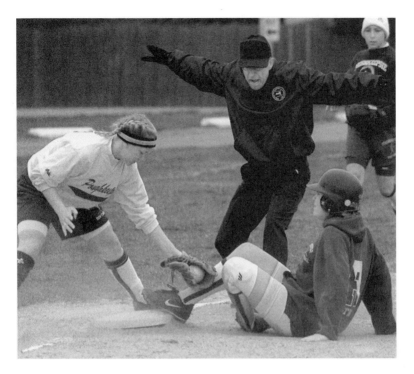

the kid has put it behind him. Immediately after the game, when the disappointment is still fresh, talk with your kid about winning and losing and new opportunities ahead. Ask, "What are you feeling? Why are you feeling like that?" Congratulate him for having such passion. Encourage him to maintain his composure. Help him to see that, whether a win or a loss, every game is an opportunity for learning and improvement.

■ ■ ■

WHEN YOU LOSE, PEOPLE WILL TELL YOU THAT YOU'RE A LOSER, and when you win, they'll tell you that you're a winner. Neither is necessarily true. It goes much deeper than that. You are a winner when you win well or lose in a manner that shows good sportsmanship and character — and you learn from your experience whatever the outcome. You are a loser if you win or lose poorly and learn nothing from either experience.

It's important to try to win, but winning doesn't make a winner. It's important to try not to lose, but losing doesn't make a loser. It is your response to winning and losing that makes you a winner or a loser.

Here's a true story that proves that winners can be losers and losers can be winners. When my friend's son T.J. was six years old, he played in a flag-football league. He and his teammates played with great enthusiasm, although they weren't very good. However, they were also at a great disadvantage — they kept playing teams that had cut their flags short so that they were much harder to grab. It started with just one team, but when other teams in the league saw that their opponents had cut their flags, they would do the same. When they came to play T.J.'s team, most teams arrived with flags that already had been shortened. One Saturday, when a team showed up with cut flags, some parents of children on T.J.'s team suggested that they cut their flags, too. T.J. protested, saying, "That's not right. Just because they broke the rules doesn't mean we should, too." The other kids agreed. So they didn't do it, and they lost again. The same thing happened the following week with another team, and again the following week, and throughout the entire season. They lost every game but one. The kids were extremely frustrated, but they still refused to play with illegal flags in order to "even the playing field."

> *We learn more about ourselves after our losses than after our wins.*

Then something amazing happened: Justice prevailed. At the end of the season, when it came time for the championship game, every team but T.J.'s and one other were disqualified for using short flags or for other infractions against league policy. So T.J.'s team got to play for the championship. They were beaten by the only other team that used legal-sized flags, but they didn't mind losing to opponents that played fairly — especially since they still received a big trophy for finishing second. They were delighted and justifiably proud. How much better they must have felt coming in second than a team using illegal flags would have felt coming in first. What would be the lasting value for winning unethically versus the lasting value of losing but playing with integrity? I think we know. The big trophy given to T.J.'s team surely is a testament to those young players who lost on the scoreboard but won in all the ways that really mattered.

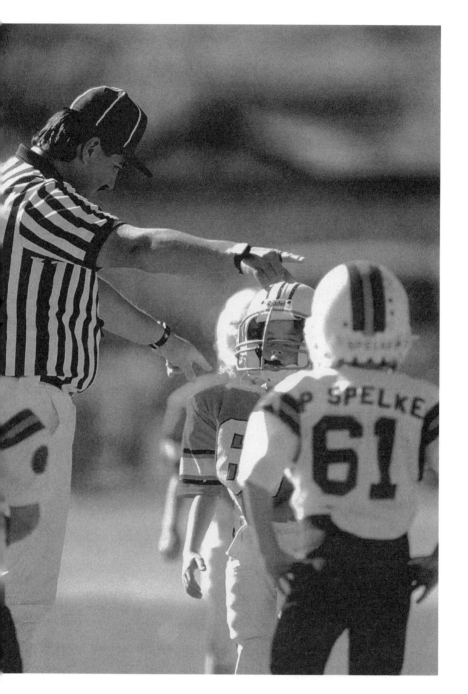

COMPETITION

My wife Connie likes to play sports for fun, without much concern for results. For example, she plays golf against the course and herself, rarely against other golfers. It drives me — the big competitor — absolutely insane! Connie doesn't fully agree with the notion that if she *competes* against another golfer, she will play better and improve her score. I myself am more inclined to agree with the likes of Venus Williams, who, after crushing the higher-ranked Jennifer Capriati in the women's tennis semifinals of the 2001 U.S. Open, told reporters, "I had a choice to play well or play badly, and I decided to step up and compete."

Such words could have motivated Connie the time she was playing in a coed squash tournament. She won her first match, but I could tell she was tanking the next one against a male opponent. I went up to her and asked, "What are you doing? You're not trying to win this match." She replied sheepishly, "Well, I feel bad about beating him." I said, with tongue firmly in cheek, "Fine. Let him go on believing he can't be beat by a woman." She gave me The Look, which meant I'd taken it a little too far, so I hurriedly sealed my lips, retreated to the seats, and started cheering her on.

Connie knew that I was only kidding. She knows how I feel about competition. I wasn't asking her to win; I was nudging her to *try to win* by competing as hard as she could. It's the same thing I ask of young athletes.

Connie did come back and win.

■ ■ ■

IN EVERY ARENA OF LIFE, INCLUDING SPORTS, THERE ARE GOING TO be ripples in the water, obstacles, challenges. Learning how to compete properly is one way to keep us moving forward in times of adversity. When I joined Athletes-in-Action after graduating from college, I went directly from a winning college program to an amateur basketball team that had a dismal 10-25 record in my first year. I had never faced that kind of adversity, where I was part of a rebuilding program.

Competing is an acquired skill.

Losing can badly affect the way a team prepares for games, but our coach, Rle (pronounced like Arlie) Nichols, refused to send us onto the floor without being ready to give our best. He made us compete *every* night. Eventually we turned things around and defeated such college powerhouses as Syracuse, UNLV (the University of Nevada at Las Vegas), and Maryland, as well as the mighty Russian national team. Our victories never would have been possible if our coach hadn't pushed us to play hard enough to improve, even when we knew we had little chance of winning. That was a real lesson for me.

Is competing an acquired skill? Absolutely. Some kids are a little more predisposed to it, but the key people in any child's life should be able to teach him or her the value of competition at a very young age. Unfortunately, many parents need a good lesson in competition themselves. If Mom came from a family that frowned on girls playing sports, she may not have experienced athletic competition first-hand. Dad, on the other hand, may have run track or been a fullback in college but never played in organized youth sports. So here are parents with two totally different perspectives: Dad thinks he understands competition but is concerned mostly with what's on the scoreboard; Mom thinks it's ill-mannered to be competitive and just hopes you're having fun playing with your friends. So if you're their kid, when you walk in the door, Mom asks "Oh, did you have a game today?" and Dad demands, "Did you win?"

"Good competition" is a complex concept, but moms, dads, coaches, and players all need to understand it. Through good competition, kids expose themselves to challenges and learn a great deal about themselves and what makes them tick. They find out what they are willing to do and what they are not willing to do to improve or to reach a goal. They learn about their physical, emotional, and mental limits.

Being competitive, win or lose, is itself a positive experience, if channeled correctly. When young athletes compete, they learn that adversity can bring them to new levels of performance. They see that hard work combined with passion really does yield results. They realize that they must take risks — try to win, set a new goal, or match up against a stronger player — in order to succeed. When they take a risk and fail, a healthy sense of competitiveness urges them to try again.

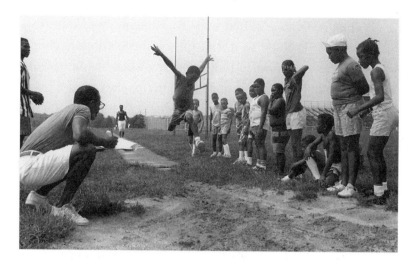

A young athlete's reactions to tough game situations will tell people what kind of competitor she is. She could find herself with one minute left in a close game against a tough team or in a blowout against a terrible team. The referee could make a bad call against her, or another player could taunt her. Will she let the situation steal her focus, or will she be able to shrug it off?

There are times when we all want to quit, when we feel we can't go another step. But what we can teach kids, through sports, is that with a little extra effort they can compete right through that quitting point. One of the best competitors I've ever had the pleasure of coaching was Seth Mehr, the player who wrote to me, saying, "Medical school is hard, but what prepared me for it the most, even more than my organic chemistry lab, was the basketball program." On our basketball team, Seth had the character to compete rather than quit when the odds were against him, and that carried over into his medical career.

Having quality competitors is every coach's dream. A quality competitor plays with passion and carries himself like a winner — with pride, humility, and composure. In a game situation, competitive spirit can make a real difference; someone who understands how to compete can prevail against someone who has greater skills but isn't a good competitor. And a good, healthy, competitive spirit is infectious. When the best players on a team are also quality competitors, great things can happen.

In 1997, my Williams team went to the Division III Final Four. We weren't better athletically than the two teams we beat to get there, but we were mentally tougher. My players understood what it meant to compete better than our opponents did. Before games, we talked about playing every possession as a competitive entity. If we could string those possessions together, we could succeed. And we did.

Jimmy Frew was the point guard on that 1997 team. Looking at him, you wouldn't think that he was very athletic. In fact, we'd kid him for walking flat-footed like a duck. But Jimmy was a tremendous competitor. We played Stockton State from New Jersey in the Sweet Sixteen, and they had a terrific guard who was chewing us up. The player who was defending him couldn't do anything to stop him. I then asked Jimmy to guard him. I told him, "You're going to have to really compete, because he's going to make you look really bad a few times. Even if we win, you're going to be razzed about it by the other guys on the team. But what I want from you is for that guy's legs to be gone by the time there's only five minutes left in the game. And another thing — *you* aren't allowed to get tired."

Jimmy got in the kid's face, but he still buried his first three shots. Jimmy looked at me helplessly, and I shrugged. I reminded him, "You have to compete on *every* possession." Jimmy did just that. In the second half he yelled to me as he ran by the bench,

"Coach, he's getting tired!" When fatigue sets in, skill level drops, and sure enough, Jimmy's man missed his last five or six shots, and we won.

We saw some great competition that night. Jimmy put out a real high-quality effort, not knowing whether it would have an effect but certain that he would not be the one reaping the glory after the game. He played hard because that's what the team needed from him; if the star player on the other team hadn't been worn down, we'd have had no hope of winning. His story shows us what it takes to be an outstanding competitor: You play hard because that's what makes you proud of your game. You don't know if your effort will make the difference, but you do know that without your effort, you won't ever be successful.

Of course, Jimmy was a mature, twenty-two-year-old college player. Can young kids compete with the same enthusiasm and wise perspective that he had? Absolutely! That's one reason why we want them involved in sports — to give them the experience of passion (fun) and struggle (work) coming together to create results that they can be proud of. But kids won't realize on their own that this is the true teaching of competition; parents and coaches must constantly remind them of it, on and off the playing field.

■ ■ ■

IN ADDITION TO LEARNING TO PLAY HARD ON EVERY POSSESSION, the good competitor must learn to rise above the natural ebb and flow of games. This is a great lesson for kids, most of whom are still learning how to handle their emotions. Many games are like roller coaster rides: You score seven straight points and feel like you're on a roll, then the other team comes back and scores eight straight points and you feel deflated, and so on. A good competitor maintains control of his own emotional situation throughout the game and exudes a sense of composure to his teammates, opponents, and fans.

Before critical road games, I would tell my team in the locker room, "When they score or you throw the ball away, the fans will go crazy. But you have to stay under control. Don't let the crowd take you out of the game."

That was advice we needed when we played a big road game against Springfield College in the NCAA tournament. We had a wonderful first half and were up by seven points before they hit a 55-foot three-pointer with a second left in the half. The fans went crazy. The first three rows ran out onto the court and did push-ups. It was wild. We went to the locker room, and I told my players, "We did exactly what we wanted to do, and we withstood their best shot. At the beginning of the second half, we have to expect them to do it again. Don't let it beat you — keep your heads." Sure enough, in the second half Springfield had a good run that concluded with a big dunk. But our team acted like it was a layup and came right back. My players knew how to compete, and they understood that winning required composure. We ended up playing one of the best games we had ever played.

The quality of the way you compete influences the quality of your play.

■ ■ ■

MOST SPORTS LEND THEMSELVES TO COMPETING AGAINST YOURSELF, which can help you improve your skill level. However, competition against another player or another team gives you a better measuring stick and greater motivation to improve. A young bas-ketball player can say, "I've practiced a lot, so I know I can knock down the 15-footer." But if he's playing another team, and the player guarding him is so quick that he can't get off that shot cleanly, he has to step up and *compete* to get that shot. It's very different from playing alone or in a noncompetitive situation. The opposing player is a competitive challenge.

We must teach our young athletes to compete until the last second ticks off the clock, because it's the competitive challenge that allows a game to be a learning experience. The variable is in what players are competing for. If a basketball team is in a close game, then of course the competitive challenge is to win. But if the team has a gigantic lead, then perhaps the competitive chal-lenge is for second-stringers to come off the bench and play well. Or perhaps the competitive challenge is for the team not to run fast breaks but to perfect their set plays, make excellent passes, and take the first natural shot.

Even when they have a big lead, coaches should never tell kids not to try to score. Don't insult the other team by not com-peting against them. If I ever heard the opposing coach tell his team to hold the ball because they had a big lead, I'd be embar-rassed. No, *compete* against my kids! I don't care if we lose by 21 or 61. Just don't insult us by not competing.

■　■　■

WHEN YOU COMPETE IN CONTACT SPORTS, YOU MUST BE PHYSICAL. Some sports, such as football, rugby, and ice hockey, require more visible aggressiveness than others, but all sports fans can appreciate tough competitors. I once coached a great kid named Brendon McGuire, whom I recruited out of Regis High School in New York. He was 6'4" and about 170 pounds when he arrived at Williams and, after spending much time in the weight room, graduated at 215 pounds. A friend asked me who played center for me, and I told him about Brendon, saying he was a strong kid but "a little soft." The team reached the Sweet Sixteen that year, and my buddy came and watched us play. After the game he asked, "Is the McGuire kid the one you said was soft?" I said, "Yeah. Don't you agree?" He said incredulously, "Harry, he's the most physical kid I've ever seen! That kid is a warrior!" I was taken aback. I realized that I had watched Brendon play every day but had seen only his shortcomings. He'd become a tremendous competitor without my noticing. At 170 skinny pounds, he'd had to fight every day of practice just to make a space for himself on the team, and through the process he'd learned to *compete*. He was a warrior, just like my friend said. The lesson? That sometimes it's helpful for parents and coaches to see their kids through other people's eyes. The point? That you don't see "competitiveness" in the scoring columns. You see it in the way a player hustles, puts his body on the line, and exhibits a will to win.

Far too many young kids don't know how to compete. Some will do anything to win and get called bad sports; others don't want to push themselves or anyone else and get called slackers. But these kids are neither bad sports nor slackers; they just haven't learned how to compete in the appropriate way. To put such boys and girls on the path to a proper perspective on how to play a sport is one of the most positive things you can do as a coach or a parent. And managing to do that successfully, to see your kid out there competing with both grace and intensity, is a thrilling experience.

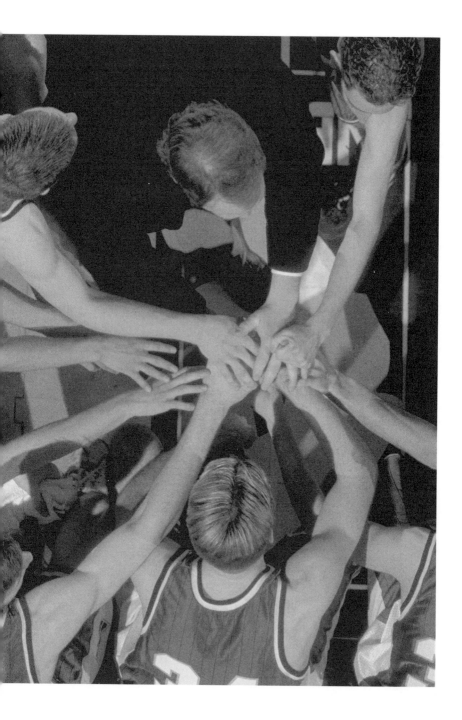

SPORTSMANSHIP & CHARACTER

Athletes should always try to win, but there's a fine line between competing hard and being immature and out of control. If kids' competitive instincts are focused primarily on the experience of playing a sport well as a team, they tend to mature quickly and develop a strong sense of character. However, kids who are allowed to focus exclusively on personal results often reveal poor sportsmanship and a lack of character.

Young athletes can be extremely competitive and, at the same time, responsible and accountable for their actions. After a victory, they can carry themselves with dignity, holding heads high and firm hands out to shake with the opposition. If they lose, they should act in exactly the same manner. Whatever the outcome of a game, players have an obligation to themselves, as well as their parents, teammates, coaches, referees, fans, schools or leagues, sponsors, and opponents, to behave appropriately.

Good competitors play hard; throughout the game, they show respect for all participants, and after the game, they shake hands with the opposition. There should be no taunting, bad-mouthing, or cursing. No complaining to or about referees. No orchestrated mugging for the camera or crowd. It's a sad state of affairs when we are surprised to see good sportsmanship out on the field. What does that say about the character of our athletes?

■ ■ ■

GOOD SPORTSMANSHIP IS REACTING TO A CRITICAL SITUATION IN A manner that builds up yourself and your team in a positive way. Bad sportsmanship is an inability to cope with emotions brought out in a tough, stressful situation. Think about it. When kids haven't been taught to put winning and losing into proper perspective, and they consider every game a do-or-die situation, their competitiveness manifests as bad sportsmanship. Some of that is human nature; we all have the potential to become a knucklehead in a competitive situation. Unfortunately, too much of it is learned from coaches, parents, and peers.

If an attitude that fosters sportsmanship isn't found at home, it certainly won't be found in the kid. Savvy parents know that focusing only on winning teaches their kids the wrong lessons about sports. But if the emphasis is not on winning, what *is* it on? Too few parents have consciously prioritized what they *should* emphasisize in order to teach their kids the *right* lessons. Even if they refrain from emphasizing winning, many parents insist that their child be made a starter or get more playing time, and they criticize the coach when that doesn't happen. Far too few support the coach if they don't agree with his methodology.

It's important to step back and make a realistic appraisal of your child's abilities and your attitude. Remember that there are many ways to win, and a coach's methodology often depends on the players he is working with in a particular season. The game plan that is best for the team this year may not yield as much playing time for your child as you would like. Instead of criticizing the coach's decision, encourage your youngster to maintain a good attitude. By telling their child, "You should be playing more, but the coach doesn't like you and is being unfair," parents give their child a crutch — "When something happens that I don't like, it's not my fault and it's not fair" — that, if not corrected, will become a habit for the rest of his life.

When a young athlete comes home from a game, the first questions that come out of a parent's mouth are what the child will assume are the most important. What are the first three questions a parent should ask?

1. Did you have fun?
2. What do you remember about the game?
3. Now what are you going to work on?

What are the first three questions a parent will be tempted to ask first but should save for later?

1. Did you win?
2. How did you play?
3. How much did your coach play you?

These two sets of questions send very different messages to the child, and the order in which they are asked tells a lot about the people who ask them. So pay attention to what you say, Mom and Dad. Your children are listening.

I HEARD SOMEONE SAY, "CHARACTER IS WHAT WE ARE WHEN NO one is looking." With my players I take it further, telling them, "Character is what you are when *I* am not looking." On my teams, I want *people of character,* not *characters.* What is it to have character? People of character have a good work ethic, are willing to sacrifice as an individual for the good of a group, compete hard but at all times exhibit good sportsmanship and integrity, and feel proud but humble in both victory and defeat. And that's just the beginning.

Character-building can be one of the primary goals of sports. Athletes who must work hard day after day to achieve personal and team goals can really learn the value of character. As one of my coaches once told me, "Character is perseverance after the initial excitement has worn off." This statement hit home for me, because I, as a player and a coach, have always held a strong belief in the importance of practice. At the first day of practice, everyone is there early, and they're pleading, "Let's go, let's go!" A couple of days later, they kind of drag in. When you've been through ten two-hour practices, your legs are dead, your back aches, you have a pulled hamstring muscle, and you worry that you're losing your position because you're not shooting well. But you know you have to keep going because that's the only way to improve. As one of my players said, "Character is crashing through the quitting point."

Going against conventional wisdom, the late famed sportswriter Heywood Hale Broun contended, "Sports doesn't build character; it reveals it." Former UCLA coach John Wooden agreed, saying that teachers and parents are the only people who can help build a child's character. Well, I think coaches are

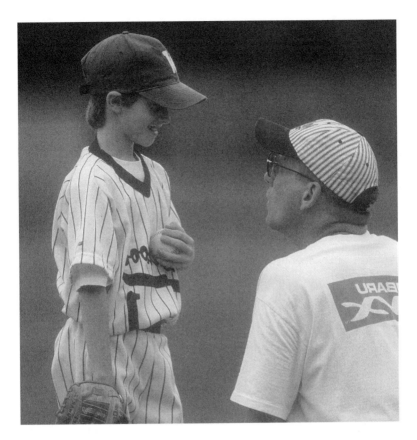

teachers — Wooden definitely was — and I believe that sports both reveals *and* builds character. I have seen so many instances in which participation in sports has benefited a young athlete in significant character-building ways. The younger the child is, the better the chance of this happening. In fact, the most formative years for kids involved in athletics are from the time they're knee-high to the age of twelve or thirteen. Even so, it's never too late. I've seen many college players unlearn poor lessons they had absorbed at an early age and develop good character and sportsmanship, even in their early twenties.

For example, in the late 1980s I had a player named Bill Melchioni whose father had been an All-American at Villanova and played with the 76ers and the Nets. Bill visited our campus as a high-schooler, and afterward one of the players he met told me, "Don't recruit Bill. He's not a good fit here. He won't do what we do, and he won't work as hard as we want." Having gotten one thumbs-down, I called the kid who had hosted Bill during his stay and asked what he thought. He said, "Coach, I think you should recruit Bill. His main problem is just that he's young." I respected both kids' opinions, but I went along with the second one because there was something about Bill that I liked. Indeed, he was undisciplined and had a spotty work ethic. Although he always played hard in games, he didn't practice hard. In fact, once I turned around in practice only to see him trying to drop-kick the ball into the basket. While Bill wasn't someone who cheated or was a bad sport, there was an edge to the way he competed. I would urge him to pull back, and I, my coaches, and our players inundated him with our ideas on what he needed to do and how he needed to think in order to fit into our program. Bill was a quality kid, and with our encouragement he continued to develop a very strong sense of sportsmanship and character. He really blossomed as a junior and developed into a team leader. He ended up being a two-time All-Conference player and a life-long friend who still is clearly proud of the lessons he learned in our program.

> No game is won or lost on just one play.

For sports to build character, coaches must teach core values that will hold true in all aspects of life, and parents must support them. Every team — youth, high school, college, or even professional — should have clearly stated core values that are intrinsic to its program. For instance, being on time was always an issue on my teams. If I was going to get only fifteen hours a week with my student-athletes, it was important that they showed respect to all their coaches and teammates by being on time. If a core value on a youth team is looking presentable, then parents should make sure that their kid tucks in his shirt and keeps his shoes tied.

A coach's core values have to be real or the kids won't buy into them. "Do as I say, not as I do" will never hold water with a young athlete. Youth, high school, and college coaches must be accountable to their players, so they'd better believe in — and live — the core values they teach. They would never again have the respect of their players if their kids saw them not following their own rules of conduct. If a coach tells his kids to be on time, to work hard, and to look each other in the eye when they speak to one another, the coach should do exactly that. If players are ready to start practice at 4:00 P.M., the coach shouldn't turn up at 4:05. If he tells his kids not to lose their tempers, then he must hold his in check as well.

■　■　■

IN MY FIRST YEAR OF COACHING AT WILLIAMS, I HAD A VERY GOOD player whom I respected except in one regard, which I discovered pretty quickly. We won our second game of the season by twenty points, but afterward he was in the shower crying. And I'm thinking, "Did we lose by twenty?" No, he was just upset because he played only half the game in the blowout and didn't score as many points as he'd hoped. Clearly he was someone who had always been asked the instant he got home,

"How many points did you score?" He had to learn to be a good teammate. When his team is that far ahead, he should be happy that all the kids who are busting their rear ends every day in practice get a chance to play.

It was my father who taught me the core value of exhibiting good sporstmanship toward my own teammates. When I was a teenager, I played Babe Ruth baseball. One day I wasn't starting, so I was sitting in the dugout doing the old legs-out, feet-crossed, hat-over-the-eyes routine. My father tapped on the side of the dugout and said sternly, "Get in the car." I went with him and soon found out why he was perturbed with me. He said, "Harry, if you're going to play on that team, you're going to look out at the field and root for your teammates." All I could do was gulp. He continued, "You decide whether you're going to go to the next game or not, because I am not going to watch you act like that. It's not right." I was thirteen or fourteen at the time, and I have never forgotten that incident. My father's words spoke volumes to me about the connection between being a good teammate and having character. Sometimes you simply have to swallow your pride and support the other guys.

■ ■ ■

YOUNG PLAYERS OFTEN HAVE TEMPER TANTRUMS WHEN THEY don't come through in a clutch situation, have a call go against them, or encounter something else that doesn't go their way, even in practice. Some youngsters simply haven't learned to control themselves during times of emotional stress. For others, temper tantrums are a way to get attention. Parents can help their kids deal with temper by emphasizing that good sportsmanship includes controlling negative emotions and teaching them to view the court, field, or rink as a classroom. Then their demeanor will be more civil, and real learning will take place.

It's not difficult for a coach to control an athlete's temper. You simply say, "You're going to sit down now, and you'll go back in when I think you're ready. If you go back in and have another temper tantrum, you will sit down again." At some point, the player will say to himself, "Gee, every time I blow my lid, I don't play." This simple technique is incredibly effective. It works best if you warn your kids throughout the season that you will remove them from the game if they act inappropriately. Of course, once you set such a rule, you have to follow through with it in all circumstances, even if the kid throwing the tantrum is the star of your team and you're trailing by one point with ten seconds left. Otherwise you're delivering an incredibly bad message to him and all his teammates.

Good sportsmanship is reacting to a critical situation in a manner that builds up yourself and your team in a positive way.

It's really important for coaches — youth-league coaches, especially — to think this through ahead of time. A competitive game can bring out a lot of emotions in a young athlete, and you have to be prepared to handle them. If a kid blows up and you aren't prepared, chances are that you will react angrily, when it's a time to teach instead. Then the young boy or girl will go home thinking, "My coach doesn't like me," instead of being on the road to learning to control temper and show good sportsmanship.

If you're the parent of a kid who throws tantrums during games or practices, it's important that you work together with the coach to help your child. At home, use goal-setting techniques. Make keeping his cool and being a good encourager of his teammates your child's goals, and talk with him about them before every game or practice. Tell your kid's coach about these new goals, and ask him to pull the kid from the game or practice if he does throw a tantrum, and not to put him back in until he regains control of himself.

> *Bad sportsmanship is an inability to cope with emotions brought out in a tough, stressful situation.*

Temperamental kids (who are much different from high-spirited kids) can be very hard to handle. I've had kids at my basketball camps who have been nightmares. Then I'd see their dads play in a senior men's league game — oh, my gosh! The apple doesn't fall far from the tree. In many cases, when I meet the parents, I realize why the kid was so difficult to work with. Of course, I've also seen many players who really have it together, and almost without exception, their parents have it together, too.

Recently I read a news story about the aftermath of an all-star soccer game. The father of one of the kids pushed one of the young players on the opposing team, a fourteen-year-old who was, allegedly, taunting the parents of the other team. When the father retaliated, it led to an all-out brawl all over the field. Think about how absurd that is. When an adult feels that he should push a fourteen-year-old who's been taunting him, then we as a society have lost — that's the definition of *losing* right there. We have lost our sense of civility, of what is right and what is wrong. And this stuff happens every day! If adults don't act like adults, is it fair that we expect our kids to learn about character and sportsmanship from us?

It's shocking to me how often we hear of violent situations involving parents, youngsters, and referees. Referees have to endure frightening abuse, including insults, threats, and even physical violence. I've seen some games in which I think the referees would be justified to sue for harassment and abuse. And I'm disgusted at the language used by coaches, kids, and parents, even at Little League games. My dad once happened to hear something pop out of my mouth that shouldn't have. He said, "Harry, I have to tell you, profanity is a small mind struggling to express itself." That lesson stuck with me. I do not allow profanity on the court, at any time, and neither should any coach or parent.

The sportsmanship of fans at all levels is of great concern. Some of the good-natured razzing that comes out of the stands from kids is creative and funny, but too much is shockingly mean-spirited. Remember that despicable incident a few years ago when fans of a rival school taunted University of Arizona player Steve Kerr about the recent killing of his father? Our country values free speech, but the right to free speech doesn't justify abusive behavior. Just because you have the right to do something doesn't mean that it's the right thing to do. Fans have as much obligation as the players to behave with character. I'm glad that the Pac-10 conference, to which Arizona belongs, is now running a sportsmanship program for its member schools.

Another worrisome form of bad sportsmanship is sulking on the part of players and coaches when they feel they are the

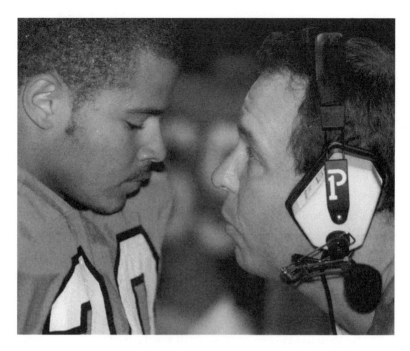

victims of bad calls. Officials cannot possibly be perfect, any more than players can, and they *will* make bad calls. It's particularly hard for youngsters to accept this, especially when those bad calls come at critical moments in a game. But all players, parents, and coaches should understand that no game is won or lost on just one play and that the first possession is every bit as important as the last possession. Don't blame the officials for a loss. I can't remember one game a referee cost me in seventeen years. We all have had bad calls go against us, but as coaches and players we often don't recognize when we've gotten the breaks at other times. A great example is the time my team had three or four calls in a row against us, and an assistant coach griped, "We're just getting robbed by the referees tonight!" I checked our statistics, then asked, "Coach, do you realize that we've taken thirty-four free throws tonight, and the other team has taken only nine?"

If a team is having trouble on the scoreboard, it's natural to look for a reason other than its own play. Therefore, it's vital that coaches and parents reinforce in young players the idea that referees are never responsible for losses. Players must be taught to accept responsibility for bad outcomes just as they take credit for good outcomes.

■ ■ ■

THERE ARE MANY VARIABLES IN THE AREA OF SPORTSMANSHIP: coaches, teammates, parents, opponents, fans, and so on. There are so many places where it can go bad. With parents and peers giving young kids little reason to think in terms of good sportsmanship, it is often up to the coaches. However, many coaches also let down the kids; many could themselves use a class in sportsmanship. Coaches run up scores, sometimes to let a player reach a milestone like scoring fifty or even one hundred points in a game. They yell at players not only on their own team but also on the opposing team, even when they are on the free throw line, in the batter's box, or lining up penalty kicks or field goal attempts. Worst of all, some employ unethical means to score and win.

I recall the time Dick Farley, the football coach at Williams College, was upset after losing a game 7-0 on a play that was technically legal but somewhat unethical. The opposing coach had devised a pass play in which the receiver hid near the sidelines, arms folded and eyes directed to the side, acting like he wasn't even in the game. When the ball was hiked, he suddenly darted into the end zone unguarded and caught the game-winning pass. The play was very underhanded, but the most important thing to me was what the ninety kids on the two teams felt about how the outcome of the game was decided. Is that how we want to teach our players to succeed?

In one basketball game that I remember well, my team committed a foul on a poor free throw shooter, but the referee called out the wrong jersey number, and the opposing coach allowed a better shooter to be sent to the line. To this day I don't know if the coach knew what he did, but I did say something about it to him after the game. If the kids on his team knew it and said nothing to him, it was just as wrong. I told my players, "Guys, we won the game and I feel great about it, but let's go over something that happened that I don't want us to be involved in.

> *Profanity is a small mind struggling to express itself.*

They sent the wrong free throw shooter to the line, possibly because he was better than the kid who was fouled. There is a school of thought out there that thinks that what they did was cute and clever. I do not. If they did it on purpose, that's cheating, and that is something we as a team will never do."

What if the situation were reversed and we were the team to benefit? I would say the same thing. In one NCAA tournament game at Springfield College, the referee was going to send our star Michael Nogelo to the free throw line. I yelled to the referee that it wasn't Michael who was fouled but another player, who was a worse foul shooter. I didn't want to win that way, and I didn't want Michael to think that I knew it was another player who had been fouled yet didn't try to do something about it. The bottom line: If we lose the game because we didn't switch free throw shooters illegally, then we should lose the game.

In another game, the officials were going to let Michael shoot free throws after a non-shooting foul, but I told them that he shouldn't be sent to the line because we weren't yet in a one-and-one situation. Such things make an impression. My players thought that I did exactly the right thing by pointing out the mistake. It's not that I wanted them to think of me as "Mr. Character," but I wanted to represent to them the consistent core values of our program. I didn't want someone on the bench to be contemplating, "I wonder what Coach is going to do this time. Because sometimes he will do this and other times he will do that. . . . If we're up twenty points late in the game, he wouldn't bother, but if we were tied, he might . . ." I wanted my kids to know exactly what I'd do, no matter the circumstance — and what I would expect them to do in my place.

When I send my players out into the world, I want them to think back on their sports experiences when they get into a sticky situation with a lot of ethical gray areas. I want them to know how I would react in their place and how I hope they would react. And I want them to know that there is a group of people out there — their former teammates — who think that's the right way to do it. At that crucial moment I want them to reveal, through their decisions and actions, the sterling character that together we helped develop years ago in our basketball program. Because character never hibernates. It builds and builds until it becomes a way of life.

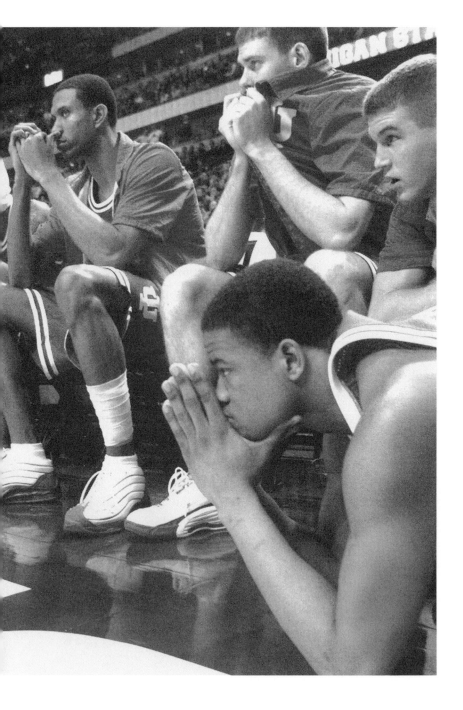

HUMILITY

My first varsity basketball coach at Williams College in 1972 was Al Shaw, who had coached my dad on his first team about twenty-five years earlier. In my third game, I scored twenty-eight points in a narrow loss to Tufts University and was sure Coach Shaw was as impressed with me as he had been with my father. To confirm this, I paid him a visit. I hoped Coach Shaw would agree with me that I was the star of the game. When he wasn't swift with the praise, I decided to remind him how many, many points I'd scored. This is when I learned the Al Shaw system for evaluating and *de*valuating performances. He looked at me and said coolly, "Harry, you did score twenty-eight points, but your man had twenty points, his sub had four, and his sub had four. That also equals twenty-eight points. So you got *nothing*. It was a wash."

Wow! That was an eye-opener for me. Slipping out of his office, tail between my legs, what did I come away with? I had come to the realization that you can't boast about your offense if your defense is lacking, and that nobody wants to hear about how many points you scored after a loss. Unfortunately, I was smart enough then only to figure out when it was proper to keep my mouth shut. What should have been a lesson in humility was, because of my neediness, no more than a humbling experience.

However, that particular lesson was only one year away. Coach Shaw retired after my sophomore year, and as of my junior year the team had a new coach, Curt Tong. I came to think of Coach Tong as my mentor and, needy as ever, would often drop into his office between classes. Once, after a win in which I thought I'd played exceedingly well, I stopped by to talk with Coach Tong about how well I'd played. I remember saying, "You know, Coach, I've been thinking that I played really well yesterday and I'm really coming along." The gist was, "Coach, please tell that me I'm good." Coach Tong was a measured guy, and he just sat there as I kept talking and talking, fishing for compliments. He finally took a deep breath, his eyes showing disappointment, and said quietly, "You know, Harry, if you're really good, you won't have to tell anybody."

> *If you have to tell people that you're good, it implies that they haven't arrived at that conclusion on their own.*

We laughed, but it was like I'd been cut with a knife. Believe me, I heard that.

I remember going back to my dorm room and sitting on the edge of my bed and just thinking about Coach Tong's words. Their meaning was clear: If you have to tell people that you're good, it implies that they haven't arrived at that conclusion on their own. And there is usually a good reason for that! Coach Tong's words were life-changing for me, helping me as a player then and as a coach years later. That day I learned humility first-hand and in a deeply personal way. Soon I came to understand it as an essential ingredient for players of good character, particularly in team sports.

■ ■ ■

I STILL THINK OF COACH TONG'S WORDS WHEN I TURN ON THE television and see a football player score a touchdown and do a jitterbug in the end zone or sack a quarterback and beat his own chest for the benefit of the crowd and cameras. I think of them when I see a basketball player slam-dunk the ball and then stand over the defensive player while gyrating in the direction of the opposing team's fans. The mugging for the camera, the finger pointing, the dancing, and the taunting that goes on between players is at a ridiculous, infuriating level and sends horrible messages to young sports fans in search of role models.

How much better it would be if young athletes could have seen the classy players on John Wooden's championship teams at UCLA in the 1960s and '70s. They pointed fingers only to recognize the teammates who threw the passes that led to their baskets. Parents and coaches should strongly encourage young athletes to act with that kind of class. If they score or make a great play, tell them to act not as if it were a miracle but as if it were something they did every day, and to get back to play defense. The other players and their teammates will respect them all the more for it. As Coach Tong would have said, there's no reason to tell people how good you are when they can see it for themselves.

I expected my Williams players to carry themselves like winners, which meant that they did not strut around as though they didn't believe it was possible for them to lose. As good as they were and as successful as the Williams teams they led were, Jimmy Frew and Michael Nogelo personified humility. They exhibited a confidence that was quiet rather than brash, and I respected them for it. If we had a big game coming up, I'd ask, "Are we going to win?" They could have answered, "Of course, Coach, there's no way we can lose." Instead they would tell me,

> *Humility is a realistic appraisal of who you are.*

"If we work hard, Coach. We just have to go out there and do it." That's not what a lot of coaches want to hear, but I liked it because it was realistic. It's not that Jimmy or Michael lacked confidence in the team; rather, they phrased their answers carefully because they had humility. They weren't prematurely convinced of victory. They knew they were good, but they also knew that they would accomplish nothing if they didn't work hard.

Humility keeps good, confident players from becoming overconfident or cocky. Cocky players have forgotten what it took to get where they are — hard work, practice, and discipline. That often means that they don't work as hard as they should and don't improve as much as they could. It's not uncommon for young athletes, who are still learning how to handle success, to become cocky. Thankfully, we can guarantee that every cocky young player will eventually experience defeat. Whether the defeat inspires in them a sense of humility or of bitter resentment depends, in part, on the response of their coaches and parents to that defeat. Does it become a time to mourn or a real teaching moment?

Of course, cockiness can develop not only from overconfidence but also from lack of confidence. Sometimes kids are so insecure that they feel they must convince people of how good they are. Instead of working hard to improve, they posture. My feeling is that these kids need not to be cut down to size but to be lifted up and injected with an enthusiasm for learning the game. Show them that they *can* improve, and often they *will* improve — in their skills and in their attitude.

■ ■ ■

CONTRARY TO WHAT MANY PEOPLE BELIEVE, HUMILITY IS NOT A lack of confidence, nor is it a lack of pride, nor does it mean that a person must be meek and mild-mannered. I once had a player who was a great athlete and had tremendous pride in the team but was so concerned about coming across as immodest that he seemed to apologize for every little thing, as if even talking to you were an intrusion. When he'd come into my office, he'd peek inside and say weakly, "Coach, I'm sorry I'm bothering you, I don't mean to bother you . . ." His attitude translated onto the court. He was so concerned about seeming like a ball-hog that he'd often pass up an open shot in favor of giving the ball to a teammate. Humility is not about shooting a little or a lot but about shooting when you should. That was a hard lesson for him to learn.

It is true that too much pride can destroy humility, but nowhere does it say that humility can destroy pride. Humility is not false self-deprecation but, rather, a realistic appraisal of who you are. A player who acknowledges that he is good at basketball is not bragging if he is indeed good at basketball. This is an important lesson that parents and coaches can teach kids, because it holds true in all aspects of life. Obviously, it is usually the better players — or players who overestimate their talent — who must learn humility; self-confidence, rather than humility, is generally the bigger issue for players who are not as talented as others.

Humility is integral to good teamwork. Many young players take pride in themselves but don't understand the concept of having pride in a group. One reason that it's such a long leap for them to begin taking pride in a team is that they will likely have to make sacrifices as individual players in order to help the collective. For example, a hockey player may take pride in the fact that he's a great forward and think that he should play an average of five shifts every period. But if his humility allows him to think about fitting into the team

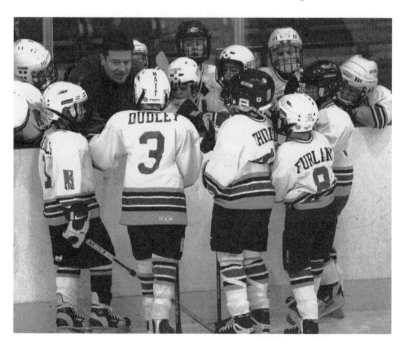

concept, he might be agreeable to playing only two shifts per period. In fact, he may be asked to sit on the bench, although he thinks he should start. If the boy is well taught and continues to be encouraged and supported by his coaches and parents, he won't have to swallow his pride but instead can redirect it toward his job as a role player (while he works hard to become a starter). He can learn to take pride in what the team is doing even though he would have arranged things differently than the coach did.

I learned from my college coaches that humility is teachable. A humble spirit may be God-given, but humility can be a learned skill. Not enough adults realize this. Parents and coaches can have a huge positive impact on kids, particularly those younger than twelve, by talking to them about the right and wrong way to conduct themselves in the sports arena and in life. I have seen many kids start to take pride in the classy way they have learned to act when they don their uniforms and represent their teams. Moreover, it is appropriate for them to take pride in the fact that they have their priorities straight. In fact, inspiring that pride should be a goal of their coaches and parents.

In sports, there are plenty of real situations with substance and drama that are exciting to watch unfold. Young athletes don't have to copy the wild, in-your-face antics they've seen on television. Much more exciting for fans to witness are real moments when humble yet enthusiastic players reveal talent but don't make a big deal of it, express passion for playing a great sport as it was meant to be played, and share emotional moments with their teammates. Kids love attention and will show off to get it, but we need to tell them that performances informed with humility are much more impressive.

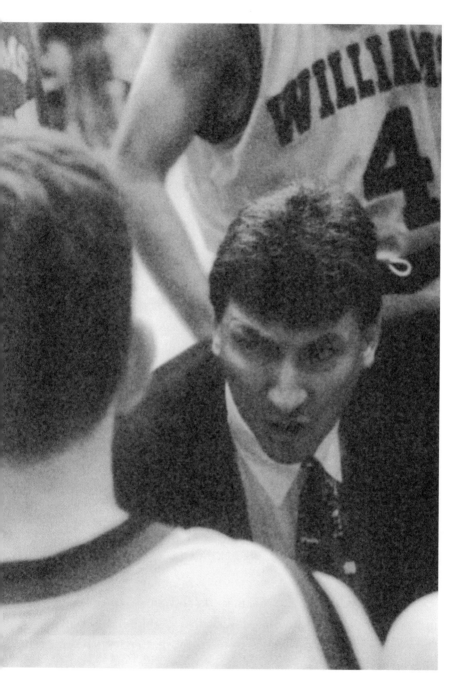

CRITICISM & PRAISE

If you participate in athletics for any length of time, then, as in most activities, eventually you will be singled out for both criticism and praise. I think my own responses to criticism and praise as a youngster were quite typical for a kid. When I was criticized, most of the time I thought it was unfair, and only occasionally did I think it was justified, but I didn't feel good about it either way. How did I feel about praise? I knew some praise I received was deserved and some was unwarranted, but the funny thing is that I felt great about it either way. Most people I know felt exactly the same way. Many adults *still* feel that way. The human ego seems to be inherently tuned to respond to the positive and negative comments of others.

Criticism is generally regarded as a pejorative word; even when it is called *constructive criticism,* we are often resistant to it. That is unfortunate, because criticism is necessary for teaching. How can you improve if you don't know what you need to work on? One of the great things about sports is that it creates in kids enough of a desire to improve that they are willing — perhaps — to hear and learn from criticism. They also begin to learn to distinguish between criticism that is constructive and criticism that is not — and how to respond in either case.

In itself, criticism is neither good nor bad; it depends on whether we learn from it or are so wounded by it that we reject it. This is a great lesson for parents and coaches to teach kids, but it is a very difficult lesson, and too few adults have learned it themselves.

■ ■ ■

BY NO MEANS SHOULD THE BURDEN OF MAKING A POSITIVE OUT OF criticism rest squarely on youngsters' shoulders. They certainly shouldn't be expected to respond favorably to their coach screaming at them, "Don't do it that way! I didn't teach you to do it like that! What are you thinking?" Unfortunately that's how most of the so-called "teaching" is done. For criticism to be helpful to young people, it must be delivered in a manner that is clear, honest, sensitive, and age-appropriate. Its purpose should be *constructive*. Even so, youngsters may be so cynical, suspicious, or thin-skinned that they will assume a coach's intention is to attack or demean rather than to teach in the best sense of the word.

One afternoon last year I watched the Williams College women's softball team play against a local rival. At an inopportune time, a batter missed a sign from the coach and struck out on the next pitch. The coach called her over and asked, "What happened there? Did you miss the sign?" When the player nodded yes, the coach went on to explain, very calmly, why it's important to pay attention to the coaches. I was impressed. But after the game I overheard that young woman talking to another player, and she was saying, "Yeah, Coach sure yelled at me for missing a sign." My only comment was: "Wow!" The coach never had yelled, and I regarded her conversation with her player as excellent teaching, yet the player's perception was strikingly different. This is a good example of how difficult it can be to communicate with kids when criticism is involved.

One year I sat down with my seniors at the end of the season and said, "I want to do a little exit interview. I want you to tell me what I need to do better." On cue, one of the seniors piped up, "Coach, you're way too critical. Your critical comments far outweigh your praise." I was taken aback, because I always considered myself to be generous with encouragement, but rather than protest, I said, "Okay, that's good to know. I'll be more aware of that from now on." The next year I wanted to find out if what he had said was true, so I brought in someone to chart my comments over the course of fifteen to twenty practices. I told him to categorize what I said to my players as Teaching Comments, Negative Criticism, Neutral Statements, and Positive Comments. When it was all done, the positive comments, or the praise, outweighed the negative criticism ten to one. But guess what — the team thought the exact opposite! It goes to show that kids hear everything you say, but they hear criticism a lot louder.

> *Encouragement is saying the right thing at the right time.*

Remembering their own youth, adults should realize that criticism carries much more weight than praise. In fact, I'd say that it takes ten positive comments to overcome the impact of just one negative comment. This is true not only for very young kids but for college athletes as well. If you tell a player that she's not hustling, not running the plays correctly, or not getting in good position, you will probably bruise her ego. That's fine — it's important for athletes to learn how to handle criticism — but be prepared to offer her praise soon afterward, and to take the time to teach her how to improve her game.

It's important not to treat everybody in the same manner. You must adapt your handling to the individual. I could have said anything to my star point guard Jimmy Frew and he would have been fine. Would it have stung a little? Yes, but he had a great deal of self-confidence and never would have gone to bed thinking he was worthless just because a coach criticized him. However, a few years later I had another point guard who was very sensitive to criticism; if I had said the same things to him that I said to Jimmy, he would have been scalded. The key for parents and coaches is to understand and work with the temperament of the individual kid. Every kid needs proper criticism, but that criticism must be delivered in a way that that particular kid will hear, so that he can learn from it.

Kids hear everything you say, but they hear criticism a lot louder.

Equally important is that criticism — from a coach, parent, or teacher — be directed at a particular behavior and not at the person. None of us ever forgets cruel words that were insensitively directed our way, in and out of sports. Like

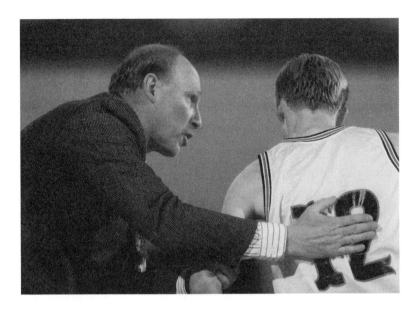

many people, I still carry around the really bad stuff, such as handing a college application form to an English teacher and having him say, "You're not good enough material for that school." Ouch! That was thirty years ago, and I remember it as if it were yesterday. I myself have made some comments to players that I really regret, and I can tell you, they certainly remember what I said. And so many times I've heard a coach yell at a child, "What are you — stupid?" That's the kind of comment that would hurt anyone, but eight-, nine-, and ten-year-olds are at such a formative stage that if they hear such criticism, they will never forget it. They will also believe it. Telling a kid he isn't running the play correctly is not the same as telling him he is stupid. Instead of becoming irate and hollering at a kid after a play was messed up, a coach should ask calmly, "Didn't we just go over what we want you to do on this play? So let's try it again that way."

Kids will mess up plays; it's inevitable. That's one reason they need coaches, isn't it? So when a young player makes a mistake, coaches and parents shouldn't act like the kid has broken one of the Ten Commandments. In fact, coaches should make sure they aren't themselves responsible for the mistake. It's a gross assumption to think that kids understand the lingo of the sport and will do exactly what they've been told without being carefully walked through the lesson. You can blow the whistle during a scrimmage of nine-year-olds and say, "Hey, you've got to *box out* in basketball," or "You have to be able to *hit-and-run* in baseball," or "You can't be *offsides* in hockey," and so on. If you then walk away without explaining what you meant, it's quite possible that eighty percent of the kids are thinking, "What's that mean? How do I do it?" And because you seemed so angry, they are afraid to ask any questions. Coaches use terms like these all the time to explain how we want something done, but we have to make sure the kids understand them. We have to be patient. We have to explain and then repeat, and maybe repeat again. That's called teaching.

■ ■ ■

COMMUNICATION BETWEEN YOUNGSTERS AND ADULTS MUST BE open and honest. In athletics, where kids' egos are often tied to their performance, good communication with the coach becomes vitally important. When coaches offer criticism to young athletes, for example, they also must explain to them how to become better, smarter players. If players venture to ask why the team employs particular plays or tactics, the last thing they need is for their coach to say, "Because it's my team, and I want you to do it that way, end of discussion." For a player to feel invested in a team concept, he or she must feel that the coach has an investment in developing the team's players.

Moreover, a coach should never change a kid's role on a team — take a kid out of the goal, the cleanup spot in the batting order, the anchor position on the relay team, and so on — without giving an explanation. It can be like a slap in the face. I once made the mistake of removing a player from the starting lineup without telling him beforehand. The ensuing announcement to the whole team in the locker room just before the game affected not only my relationship with the player but also the morale of the team.

Criticism should be directed at a particular behavior, not the person.

Sometimes a coach will change a player's role not because he's playing badly but simply because it improves the overall team strategy. However, if the coach doesn't explain the reason for the change to the athlete, the player may wrongly think that his role has been changed because he has done a poor job. Without further encouragement from the coach about his new role, the player faces an incredibly demoralizing situation.

If a player actually has been demoted because of poor performance, then it's even more important to tell him the reason for the change. It's also a great idea to remind him that if he works hard and improves, he can regain his stature on the team, if not his old position. A child shouldn't be crushed when a coach finds fault with his play, because hard work and a good attitude will lead to praise later on. Youngsters won't learn this difficult lesson unless it is taught to them by adults who have experienced it, in or out of sports.

A woman once told me that her nine-year-old son had developed a bad attitude after being replaced at the quarterback position without explanation. He assumed that the coach blamed him for the team losing its first game. In the absence of encouragement from the coach, she was able to get her son to work hard in his new role by astutely pointing out what she had learned from her own work experiences. She told him that the more positions he learned to play well, the more valuable he would be to his team.

The mother said that the reason her son listened to her is that she gave him a true appraisal of the situation, rather than babying him. She didn't say that the coach was wrong or unfair in his decision; she just told her boy to work hard and show what kind of player he was so that the coach might see things differently. She understood that coddling is nearly as bad as being hypercritical.

■ ■ ■

IT'S IMPORTANT TO SUPPORT AND ENCOURAGE CHILDREN WITHOUT coddling them. Coddling doesn't help a young person deal with the realities of a situation. Rather, it stunts growth and in no way prepares kids for the hard, realistic world they will enter when they are older. You don't want to always assure kids that everything will be hunky-dory, without any real effort or discipline on their part, and then have them begin their first job and discover that they are totally unprepared to buckle down and work or to handle workplace criticism. Parents and coaches can really help kids by telling it like it is. You'd be doing a teenage boy a disservice, for example, if you tell him that at 175 pounds he'll be an outstanding collegiate

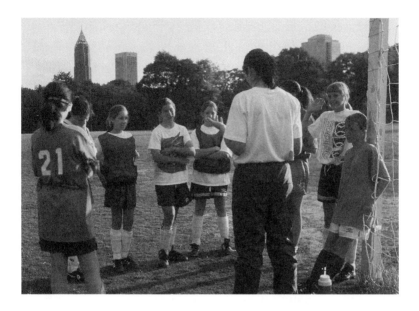

defensive lineman. You don't want to wait until after he is chewed up before advising him to consider another position or start spending a lot of time in the weight room.

It can be difficult for parents to recognize when it's the right moment to inject a dose of needed realism into their children's situation, especially when the easiest thing would be to comfort, console, and coddle them. If you have a son who is obese and he comes home every day and watches television with a cupcake in his mouth, it would be terrible parenting to tell him that he is doing a great job of exercising and is looking healthy. It's certainly not going to help him. Say you tell your daughter that if she does a good job on her homework, you'll take her to the movies Friday night. If she does her homework in a mediocre fashion and you still take her to the movies, you're not helping her. As hard as it is to disappoint your daughter, it's important to have her know what is and is not good work.

In cases like these, praise is more damaging than criticism. Adults must resist telling a child that he has done a good job, or reward him for doing a good job, when he hasn't. When I was a student, I occasionally handed in work that I knew was mediocre, but it was accepted and praised. I wish someone had just told me, "Hey, that's not good," and challenged me to do better. And I can't tell you how many times I've ended a practice by saying, "Good job!" and then asked myself, "What the heck are you saying? They weren't working as hard as you know they can. That wasn't a good job at all."

> *Coddling is nearly as bad as being hyper-critical.*

Praise is the easiest thing to say, but when used inappropriately it gives young athletes an unrealistic perception of who they are and what is the right way to act.

There's a better way for parents and coaches to help kids, and that's by asking them, "Do you want to improve? Are you willing to work to improve? If you are, I'll help you." Kids aren't perfect, and while there are some times when they need to be babied, there are other times when they really need to be told the hard truth. Balance is the key.

When kids come into my office and say, "Coach, I should be playing more," I'll say, "You have value to us because of A, B, and C. You might get more playing time if you did X, Y, and Z, but right now I don't think you've earned it." It's remarkable how positively those kids will respond to what I've said. They haven't been coddled or criticized. They have learned exactly where they stand in my eyes and, I believe, have been encouraged by hearing me say that they have immediate worth and can improve to a point where they can have more value to the team.

SOME TIME AGO I HEARD A GOOD STORY, AND IT'S STUCK WITH ME ever since. I often tell it to the audience of parents that shows up on the final afternoon of summer basketball camps to see their kids demonstrate new skills, introduce new friends, and receive their "graduation" certificates.

Let's say you were out one day and spotted a perfect little caterpillar cocoon. You might come back and visit it every day, waiting for signs of life — it's not every day that you get to see a butterfly being born. Finally the day arrives when you see the butterfly struggling to emerge from the cocoon. It struggles for a while, then rests. Shortly it resumes its struggle, then it rests again . . . struggles, then rests. You feel sorry for the little creature and run back to the house for a pair of scissors. Returning, you very carefully cut away the cocoon so that the butterfly can come out.

The butterfly at last emerges, but something's terribly wrong. It can't fly. Why? Its wings aren't strong enough. In unthinking kindness, you relieved the butterfly of its struggle to enter the world, but it needed that struggle to make its body strong enough for flight. Without that struggle, the butterfly is crippled.

In the same way, parents often open the cocoon for their kids. It can be difficult to watch your child struggling, but for the most part that struggle is imperative to growth. Without challenges to overcome and adversity to conquer, your child won't gain the inner strength necessary to take flight in the world. So when you see your child struggling, Mom and Dad, be fair and be honest. Before you run to soothe away your child's frustration, take a step back and consider the situation from an objective standpoint. Is this a moment when your child needs his or her cares lifted away? Or is this a true teaching moment, when a few honest words of encouragement and critique could help your child grow?

■ ■ ■

ENCOURAGEMENT IS SAYING THE RIGHT THING AT THE RIGHT TIME. When he was a young player breaking in with the Green Bay Packers in the early 1960s, Jerry Kramer was criticized for one entire practice by Coach Vince Lombardi. He was torn to shreds. Afterward he sat alone in the locker room with his face in his hands, thinking about quitting. Then Lombardi walked in, put his hand on his shoulder, and said, "Jerry, I think you have what it takes to become the best offensive guard in the NFL." That one perfectly timed bit of praise entirely changed Kramer's outlook, and he did go on to become the best guard in football. No young player should be subjected to the constant criticism with which the legendary coach bombarded his professional players to motivate them. But finding the right words at the right time to encourage players to new heights is a rare opportunity.

In 1997, Michael Nogelo was an All-American and our star player at Williams. (That's him with me in the photo at right, after a big game.) But I told him, "As good as you might think you are, and as great as people say you are, I will tell you when you're truly great." Michael had many outstanding games, but when we played Springfield College in a high-stakes game that would decide our standing in the NCAA tournament, Michael was atrocious. If he'd stood on a pier and tried to throw the ball into the ocean, he would have missed. With seven minutes to go, we were down by twelve points, but we soon closed the gap. At a pivotal possession, although Michael was struggling, I wanted him to shoot the ball. So we worked the ball down the court and got the ball into his hands, and Michael lined up for the shot.

If they were the best player on their team, regardless of their shooting percentage that night, ninety-nine out of one hundred kids would have taken that shot. It was what everyone expected. But Michael saw another opportunity. He fired the ball to a teammate under the basket, who laid it in. That play gave us the lead and propelled us to victory. It was an emotional game, and afterward, some of our kids were crying in the locker room. I put my arm around my star, who had gone a dismal three for nineteen, and said, "Michael, you became great tonight."

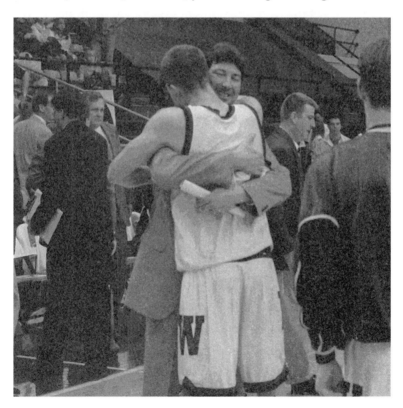

All year long, Michael had been criticized and praised with realistic appraisal. We had built an atmosphere in which our players could try and fail and not feel demoralized, so Michael wasn't hesitant. He wasn't afraid to have the ball at the critical moment, and he was prepared to make a difficult decision, without fear of the consequences. He made the right decision.

■　■　■

AT MY GIRLS BASKETBALL CAMP, WE END OUR DAY BY LETTING A few volunteers come forward and try to make baskets within five seconds in front of all the other girls. It's very informal, and the pass I throw to them might go straight up in the air or way off to the side. I always hope that the girls who aren't very good will fling it toward the basket and it will go in, because that would be a tremendous boost for them. But even after a miss, all the coaches say, "Good try," and give them high-fives, while the other campers applaud.

I must admit that I fight the urge to insist that the girls keep shooting until they make a basket. I wonder if it is appropriate that they receive praise for missing a shot, because then it doesn't really mean much when they receive the same reaction for making a basket. So why don't we change our policy and stop praising the girls after a miss? Because we don't want to discourage their budding enjoyment in playing the game, and we do want to applaud them for risking failure in front of their peers and coaches. If it's 5-4-3-2-1 and the young girl flubs an easy shot, we don't want to upset her by saying, "Ohhh, I can't believe you missed that!" We don't want to create an atmosphere in which she fears failing in front of everyone. Instead, we offer only encouragement, and when the shooters get on the bus to go home with the other girls, they start talking about other things that went on during the day and don't have any lingering embarrassment. So it's best that I bite my tongue.

Knowing when to hold your tongue and when to speak out is a challenge. I certainly don't get it right all the time; no one does. But as hard as it is for me to make that decision with the kids at my camps and my college players, it's even harder for parents, when their own kid is the one out there making mistakes. Of course you want your child to excel, and when you can see the mistakes he is making, it's natural to want to correct them. The important thing to remember is that your youngster will hear the "correction" as criticism. And when criticism is heard over and over again, or when criticism comes just at the point at which the youngster tries to stretch his abilities and fails, it's discouraging.

The question of *when* to criticize is itself answered by the question of *why* you think criticism is necessary in a particular moment. The purpose of criticism is to teach. Before you criticize, you must ask yourself: Is this a moment to teach my kid to execute correctly? Or is this a moment to support my kid's self-confidence and enthusiasm for the game?

Handling criticism positively is a difficult challenge for young athletes, as it is for all of us. The way in which we deliver it — not only our words but also our tone and timing — can make an enormous difference in the way our youngsters hear it. The question they must learn ask themselves is, "Do I wallow in it, or do I bounce?" One hopes that with encouragement from their coaches in the gym and their parents at home, they will choose to bounce.

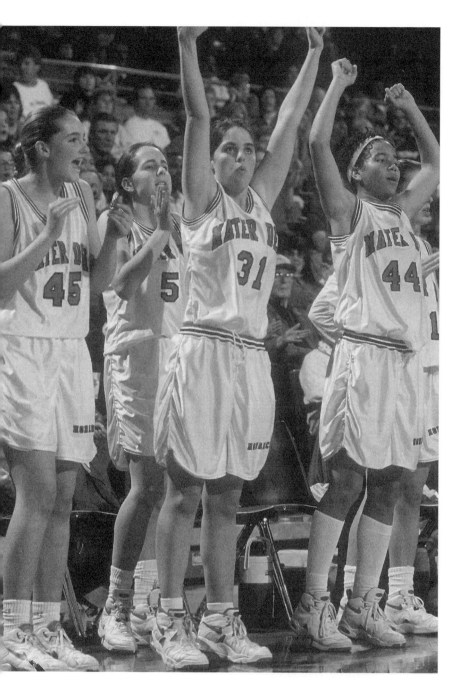

ENTHUSIASM

It was Ralph Waldo Emerson who wrote, "Nothing great was ever achieved without enthusiasm." These words, though written by someone who never homered, scored a touchdown, or ran the high hurdles, certainly hold true in sports, where disinterest sabotages work and success. Enthusiasm is a positive manifestation of passion, the catalyst for young athletes to develop a work ethic and improve their skills. While the passion that drives hard work is inspirational, enthusiasm — its high-energy, visible side — is infectious.

■ ■ ■

IN THE EARLY 1990S, I HAD A MEMORABLE PLAYER ON THE basketball team at Williams College named Robert Williams. He was described by one newspaper as the "Charles Barkley of Division III," because at 6'3" and 240 pounds, he was undersized to play power forward. He was strong, could really run and jump, could put the ball in the basket, and played big. But do you want to know the main reason I recruited him? It was because he was so enthusiastic about playing basketball. I knew that the other players would feed off him, just as the championship Los Angeles Lakers teams of the 1980s fed off the smiling Magic Johnson. Magic loved the essence of the sport, and his teammates and coaches picked up on that.

Although recruited because of his extraordinary talent, Michael Nogelo was another kid who showed up at practice ready to play. I remember one afternoon when I had the kids run "the Russian drill," which had them going up and down the court at full speed. It was an attrition drill, and one by one the weary-legged players fell behind. Finally, only Michael was left. How do you think he ended the drill? With a thunderous dunk! Everyone cheered. It was only practice, but our star showed his teammates how much effort he was willing to make when facing a challenge. He was telling them, "Basketball is something I love, and everyone will know that by the way I play it." His enthusiasm was contagious.

> *Nothing great was ever achieved without enthusiasm.*

■ ■ ■

OF COURSE, MOST YEARS I HAD A PLAYER OR TWO WHO DIDN'T have the enthusiasm to work as hard as I would have liked. Consequently, my enthusiasm for teaching them wasn't as great as it was for teaching Robert and Michael. That's human nature. We are inspired to teach by those who have a thirst to learn. There is nothing more difficult than coaching a player who has no enthusiasm. A lot of times such a kid is playing only because Mom and Dad want him to. If that's the case, his parents are doing themselves and their youngster a great disservice. I've sat down such players and said, "You don't seem to enjoy playing, you don't seem to work hard at it, you don't seem to be enthusiastic. You have to tell me why you play, because I have no idea."

"Why do you play?" is a good question to ask young athletes. They may say "Because my friends play" or "Because I'm good at it," but the best answer would be "Because it's fun." It's enjoyable to work with kids when they are having fun out there on the field, both in games and in practices; otherwise, teaching them is like pulling teeth. Similarly, when young kids have attitude problems, they steal the pleasure out of coaching. They don't understand the influence that their demeanor has on those who work with them. If kids are exuberant and excited about playing a sport, coaches, in turn, will be enthusiastic about coaching them, and parents will be more supportive of their athletic endeavor. Unfortunately, it's almost impossible to instill total enthusiasm in young athletes. They have to bring it to the table. However, parents and coaches can work to create an atmosphere in which enthusiasm is encouraged. All they need to do is take the time to point out and cheer on the natural moments when genuine heartfelt excitement is expressed.

One reason we see so little enthusiasm among young athletes these days is that the "play" has been lost from organized youth sports. Hall of Fame catcher Roy Campanella used to say that there has to be a lot of "little boy" in you to play major league baseball. If that's true for the highest rung of a

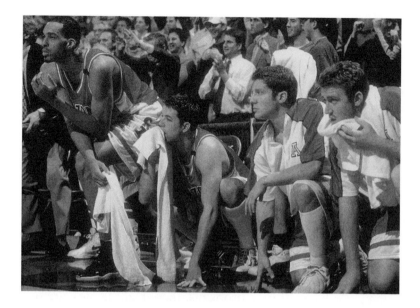

professional sport, then at amateur levels there should be even more "little boy" or "little girl" in athletes. Parents and coaches must remember that their kids are not professional athletes. They play not to get paid but because it's what they love to do.

Enthusiasm is vital for teams at practices. A player who is having a bad day shouldn't be allowed to affect the energy level of everyone else. For many years, on the first day of practice I would hand my players the rules for Williams basketball. Rule number one was "If perchance you come to practice one day and aren't enthusiastic, *pretend*." If a player came to practice after having taken a grueling exam, he'd be wrung out. But I knew that if he got involved in the activity and "acted" enthusiastic, he'd pick up the real vibes of his teammates and suddenly be up and running. It's a concept that holds true for all age levels: If you act with enthusiasm, you will become genuinely enthusiastic.

We sometimes think that the way we feel when we get out of bed in the morning is the way we'll feel all day long. But it's not true. Tell kids that they can make a choice each and every day about how they are going to approach their day, including their time spent in sports activities. They *can* make the choice to be enthusiastic.

IT WOULD BE WRONG TO SAY THAT EVERY KID ON EVERY TEAM should feel the same about the sport as everyone else on the team. Still, girls and boys need to exhibit a certain minimum level of enthusiasm, because it is the responsibility of every player to contribute to the team's collective enthusiasm. The effectiveness and strength of a team relies heavily on the collective enthusiasm of its players. All the great teams I have ever been associated with had a collective enthusiasm that was more than acceptable. Everyone could see that all the players really loved playing the game.

Matt Hunt was an All-American at Williams who just revered the game of basketball. He could not understand why every other player didn't feel exactly the way he did about such a pure, fascinating, exhilarating sport. Sometimes coaches and parents feel the same way. They can't play anymore themselves, but they want to teach the game or have their kids play so that they will understand why it is such a great game to play and watch and study. It's hard for parents and coaches who love the game to see players with good skills who don't have that passion. At

If perchance you come to practice one day and aren't enthusiastic, pretend.

lower levels of play, there's plenty of room for these players, and, in fact, they may develop that passion as they get older. But higher up the ladder, a coach may tell an unenthusiastic player that he doesn't want him on the team. Enthusiasm is essential to success. That's reality.

If I were a football coach, I wouldn't be concerned if my own children had no interest in football. It *would* bother me if they couldn't find something else to be enthusiastic about. I'd say to them, "If you don't want to play football, that's fine. But what *do* you enjoy doing?" I would want them to discover something that excites them, in or out of sports. What I've learned from my experiences is that life without passion is not *life*. Sports provides that inspiration for many kids. Others find it in music, acting, writing, painting, chess, hiking, and so on. What they do is not so important as how they do it. The most important thing we can do as parents is help our kids build enthusiasm in their lives.

■ ■ ■

FINDING SOMETHING THAT INSPIRES PASSION CAN BE A REAL challenge. Very often a child's passions match up with the things he or she is good at. Then again, a kid may have aptitude for a sport but just not be in love with the game. For example, I know a woman whose young son is a very talented baseball player but has no enthusiasm for it. He loves playing football instead. She didn't want him to give up on a sport in which he had talent; she hoped he might enjoy it more if he had different coaches or played for a different team. But she was reluctant to demand that the boy continue to play because that added pressure would have made him enjoy baseball even less.

In a case like this, parents and kids have to reach a compromise. I think back to when I was about nine and my mother wanted me to take piano lessons. I refused and refused, and she gave in. Now I would love to play the piano, and I regret that I convinced my mother to forego the lessons. Sometimes parents *do* know best, and if they feel strongly about an issue, they should acknowledge their child's concerns but not let him make the entire decision. The most reasonable way to handle such a situation, I think, is for the parent to say, "I hear that you don't want to do this, but I feel strongly that you should at least give

> *It's the responsibility of every player to contribute to the team's collective enthusiasm.*

it a chance. Let's make a deal. You try this activity for a season or a year, and if you still don't like it after that, then you don't have to do it anymore." Your child will probably grumble about it, but she may end up finding a new passion. And if she doesn't — if at the end of the designated time she still wants out — keep your end of the bargain, without protest, and let her drop it. She'll learn that you, the parent, keep your word, and that you are interested not in forcing her to do what you want but in helping her explore new opportunities. It becomes a relationship-building exercise.

If a child wants to quit a sport in which he has talent, it's important for a parent or coach to figure out why. The reason might be more complex than that he simply doesn't like the game. Perhaps the kid is turning away from the game because his coach is hypercritical. Maybe there's a family situation that's making it difficult for the kid to enjoy playing, or maybe hostile fans are making him uncomfortable. Perhaps it's even peer pressure. Kids can peer-pressure each other out of just about anything, especially enthusiasm. Just about every kid wants to be "cool," and some kids think that being too enthusiastic about a game is "uncool." When I ask questions of the girls at sports camps, it's the eight-year-olds who enthusiastically put their hands up and hope to be called on. The older girls, in contrast, start looking around at each other, because they want to make sure that volunteering an answer isn't the uncool thing to do.

Parents of teenagers have long bemoaned the power of peer pressure. Specialists in child development, I'm sure, offer many well-studied theories on the best way to insulate kids from peer pressure. But through my own experiences, I have seen that the most powerful antidote to negative peer pressure is plain and simple enthusiasm. By working with older kids to devise personal goals and encouraging their enthusiasm for reaching those goals, parents can help them rise above peer pressure and become proud of their own unique passions. Sports is one arena in which these unique passions can be developed.

■ ■ ■

ENTHUSIASM FROM PARENTS CAN REALLY HELP KIDS ENJOY SPORTS. However, parents have to be enthusiastic about the right things. Being enthusiastic over the idea of an eight-year-old becoming a Division I basketball player isn't realistic. Instead, parents should be enthusiastic about their youngster's effort, ability as a teammate, and joy in playing the game. If parents were enthusiastic about only these three things, our kids' entire focus would change for the better.

If you don't know much about the sport your child is participating in, learn it. You can't keep an open channel of communication with your youngster if you don't know the basic principles of the activity he is involved in. He won't know how to talk to you about it. When you know the game, showing interest is critical, giving support is critical, and acting with *realistic* enthusiasm is critical. Then your kid will be able to share both his positive and his negative experiences with you. However, you should recognize when it's time to back off and give your kid space, especially after a negative experience. You want to be enthusiastic about his experiences, so ask questions. But once you've gotten the answers, had a discussion, and shown your support, it might be the right time to change the subject — even if there are no problems. Emphasizing an athletic activity too much inflates its importance, making it seem more important than anything else.

> *Parents should be enthusiastic about their youngster's effort, ability as a teammate, and joy in playing the game.*

Even parents who have no background in a sport can become deeply involved in it because of their kids. For instance, a father who played football in school might become enthusiastic about girl's field hockey if his daughter plays. I know the dad of a high-school wrestler, and he's clearly a fan of the sport. I asked him if he'd wrestled in high school, and he said, "No, I just got into it because my son did. Now I really enjoy the sport." My college roommate's son is a high-school basketball player. His mother had never gone to a game until this year, and now she's a rabid fan.

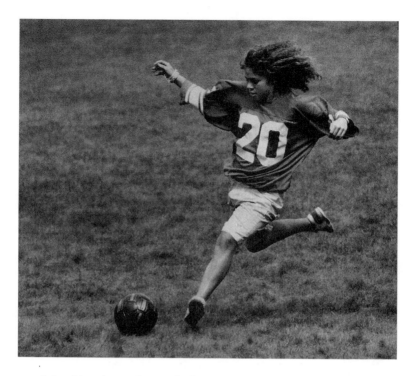

My friend Keith sends his son to golf camp, basketball camp, soccer camp, every-type camp, and he becomes involved in whatever sport his son is playing at the time. He asked me whether he should be encouraging his son to specialize in just one sport. I suggested to Keith that he allow his son to keep dabbling in different sports until he's thirteen or fourteen. Then his son can choose for himself whether he wants to focus on just one sport. I strongly believe that young kids shouldn't specialize in a single sport, as if they were already professionals. It's not necessary, and it can be harmful. Some famous athletes, like golfer Tiger Woods and tennis star Jennifer Capriati, focused on one sport from an early age. But many other famous athletes, such as basketball dynamo Michael Jordan, didn't begin to focus on a single sport until they were much older, in high school or in college. As a sports fan, I am grateful that particular sports skills become some people's full lives. These athletes are wonderful to watch, but the majority of people aren't ever going to be skilled enough to reach such heights. In fact, focusing on just one sport at an early age can harm lives, especially those of aspiring athletes who fall short of their professional ambitions and have nothing outside of sports — no skills and no plans — to fall back on.

Specialization is one of the most dangerous things we're allowing in youth sports today. We're pigeonholing kids into being enthusiastic about only certain sports, instead of all activities. Kids shouldn't worry about whether they're starring on youth teams. They should just be enthusiastic about being outside, running around, and having fun with their friends.

Unfortunately, kids, especially at a young age, tend to gravitate toward what they do well and may be really afraid of the things they don't do well. But it's important that all kids try new activities, even if they're not very good at them to start. How else will they stretch themselves and grow?

How can you encourage kids who are enthusiastic about just one sport to bring that enthusiasm to other sports and beyond? Be enthusiastic yourself. Encourage kids to test themselves in different areas. Remind them that the sport they love is only part of their lives, only part of who they are. Because the more, and more diverse, sports experiences young people have within lives that also include numerous interests and activities, the better chance they will have of being balanced and well-integrated individuals. Isn't that what we want for all our young people?

COACH SHEEHY
TALKS TO PARENTS

Youth sports seems to be facing an overwhelming national crisis of conscience. What can parents do to make a difference?

It *is* overwhelming. For a problem this large, the natural tendency is to look for a large solution. Unfortunately, I don't think that there's an easy systematic answer. If we want youth sports to be a pure, exciting, fun, educational experience, then we must make it that way in our own households and our own lives. It requires a change of heart and a change of perspective on a very individual level.

Youth sports programs put not only players but also parents in competitive situations. Our reactions to those situations stem from our reasons for getting involved in the program. It's those reasons, not the program, that need to be reevaluated. If all parents were involved in youth sports to make sure that their children had fun while learning strong values, would we have fathers killing each other when a hockey practice for ten-year-olds gets out of hand?

If we want our children to learn to handle themselves in situations of stress, then first and foremost *we* must learn to handle *our*selves. Youth sports offers us an ideal opportunity to model for our children the values that we believe are important. To get to that point, we need follow only four simple rules.

1. Take an active, participatory interest in your child's sports experience.

2. Support your child's coach.

3. Make realistic appraisals of your motivation for enrolling your child in youth sports, your child's motivation for playing, and your child's skill level.

4. Develop the healthy perspective you want your child to have. Live and speak the values that you want to instill in your child.

Do you think parents and coaches in a youth league should be accountable to an oversight board?

Oversight boards look good in books, but they can be hard to institute, and in some cases they don't make much of a difference. The problem is membership. The value of a board is tied to the philosophies of the people who are on it. Sitting on an oversight board for a youth athletic program is a big responsibility, and the people who are most likely to do it are those who have a real interest in its decisions — parents. And how many parents can be neutral or objective in decisions regarding their kids?

I'm not saying that we shouldn't have oversight boards, because for many youth sports programs they can do a lot of good, but we must openly acknowledge and guard against their potential shortcomings. It can help if the program drafts a constitution that outlines the rules by which an oversight board makes its decisions, as well as standards of conduct for coaches, players, and fans. The more specific a program can be about what is and isn't acceptable from its participants, the more useful its oversight board can be.

If a kid loses his temper during a game and his coach doesn't discipline him, what can his parents do?

It's natural for kids to feel disappointed or frustrated when the game isn't going their way, but if those emotions lead to an inappropriate comment to the referee, an altercation — physical or verbal — with the opposition, lack of support for teammates, or other displays of temper and poor sportsmanship, then discipline is necessary. One of the most important lessons of sports is how to control your emotions in a stressful situation, and if kids are allowed to have temper tantrums, they're not learning that lesson.

If your kid loses his temper during a game and his coach does not discipline him, talk to the coach. Tell him that the pressure of the game seems to be spotlighting an issue that you're working on with your kid — controlling his temper. Ask the coach to pull your kid from the game whenever he loses his temper. The coach should explain calmly to your child that negative outbursts are not acceptable and that he will have to sit on the bench until he's cooled off. The coach should also remind your kid that when he learns to control his temper, he'll be a better player and a better teammate.

At home, talk with your kid about setting two important goals: keeping his emotions under control and being a good supporter of his teammates. If your kid comes home upset because the coach pulled him from a game, don't give in to the urge to comfort him. Tell your child that you think the coach was right to pull him from the game, and repeat the lesson that the coach should have offered: Controlling your temper is an important part of being a good team player.

If a kid loses his temper during games and his coach does discipline him, should the parents still get involved? Or should they leave the discipline to the coach?

If a coach's discipline seems appropriate, parents don't need to get involved; they should simply support the coach's actions. The only time parents should get involved is when the punishment doesn't fit the crime. Let's say that a young basketball player is called for a foul, and she angrily questions the call. (Whether or not the call is correct is beside the point; young athletes should never be allowed to be rude to the referee.) In this sort of situation, the coach might call the player over to the sideline and tell her that making angry gestures toward a referee is not an acceptable behavior, and if she does it again, she will be pulled from the game.

That seems like an appropriate response from a coach. But now let's say that the player instead screams at the referee. If all the coach does is call her over to the sideline, or if the coach pulls her from the game but puts her back in ten seconds later, the coach isn't sending a strong enough message to her players about what is and isn't acceptable behavior on the court. In this situation, parents might consider speaking to the coach about instituting a firmer policy of discipline for their child.

It can be hard to come to this decision. Parents usually have a war of values going on inside them. They want their kid to play as much as possible, but they also want her to learn the right way to play. Parents who can step back from the game and think only about the values they want their kid to learn from sports are both wise and rare.

How can you tell whether a coach is being too critical?

The difference between criticism and verbal abuse can be a gray area. Some people may think that a coach who regularly yells at his players is abusive; others may not. The criticism that is appropriately directed at twenty-year-olds might be considered abuse if it were directed at eight-year-olds. I believe that real verbal abuse is something you recognize when you hear it. It's not limited to profanity but can include a coach's tone, the actions that go with the words, and the focus of the criticism. Remember: For criticism to be helpful, it must be directed at a behavior, not at a person, and it must be appropriate to the age of the individual involved.

How should a parent talk to a coach whom the parent thinks is harming a kid's athletic experience?

If you believe that the coach's interaction with your child is actually harmful and you intend to speak with him about it, be careful. Voicing your opinion about a coach's methodology is a tricky business. Sadly, most coaches hear nothing but criticism from parents and fans. If you want to make a difference for your child in a positive way, be positive with the coach. You have to assume that a coach's reasons for getting involved in youth sports match your reasons for placing your child in a youth sports program. Your goals may be slightly different, but when you break it all down, you're both coming from the same place.

What's the best way to deal with a coach who has an abrasive personality?

This situation requires more maturity on the part of parents than probably any of us possess. Some people are like that — they're simply abrasive. In other cases, their personality just doesn't mesh with yours. Some parents might be tempted to pull their kid from a team whose coach is abrasive or unpleasant. You can't really blame them; every parent wants the absolute best for their child. But what lesson does that teach kids — that they can spend their life avoiding people they don't get along with? That's just not true.

If you don't like the coach, that's fine — just don't communicate that attitude to your child. If your child doesn't like the coach, consider the situation a teaching moment. Remember the butterfly story — every kid needs challenges in order to grow and learn. Sit down with your child and talk through the situation. Don't encourage his belief that the coach is mean or that the coach hates him, but instead help him see what he can expect from this season with this particular coach — the fun experience of playing on a team as well as the maturity-inspiring experience of building a relationship with someone who is difficult to get along with.

This can be a good teaching moment for parents, too; you'll learn how to step back from a situation and analyze it from the perspective of what's best for your child, not what makes him or you most comfortable.

If the coach isn't teaching the game in the way that parents think it should be taught, should they teach kids on their own, at home?

It's great for parents to get involved in their kid's sports experiences. The danger comes when what the parents are teaching contradicts what the coach is teaching. It's not uncommon for parents to disagree with a coach's philosophy or game plan. But as long as the coach acts within the parameters of providing a sound experience, parents should not interfere. Contradicting the coach is one of the quickest ways to undermine her authority.

In no situation should you ever let your child know that you don't respect the coach. When your child thinks that the coach can't teach, she becomes unteachable, and the season becomes an educational wash. Remember: Just because a coach doesn't teach as well as you might like doesn't mean that your child can't learn from the experience of playing for her.

Remember also that there are many different ways to win, both on and off the scoreboard. A coach's philosophy may be different from your own, but as long as it emphasizes values you want your kid to learn, you should support it. It's not often that you'll come across a coach who is teaching values that you don't want your child to learn. More common is that the coach won't emphasize certain values as strongly as you would like. If that's the case, it's not inappropriate for a parent to augment — not contradict — what the coach is teaching.

How should a coach talk to a parent whom the coach thinks is harming a kid's athletic experience?

Teaching kids the *skills* of the game is a difficult science, but teaching them the *values* of the game is a true and difficult art. What's even more difficult is teaching kids whose parents don't understand the values of the game.

If a parent acts as though he has a decided plan for his kid that depends on the kid being a star player and never making a mistake, and if that parent is unjustly critical of his kid during games and practices, it's hard for a good coach not to interfere. It's absolutely unjust for a kid not to enjoy or learn solid core values from his athletic experience because of a parent. But what can you do? It's his kid, right?

This type of situation has a lot of variables, and the best way to proceed is cautiously. Be very clear with *all* the parents about what you're trying to do with the team this season. Explain both the goals the team will aim for and the core values the team will operate with. Write them down and distribute them, if you think that will make your plan clearer. Then, in the event that a parent seems to be harming his youngster's athletic experience, you can speak with him not about his "wrong" attitude but in terms of supporting the team's endeavor. Asking him — quietly and carefully — to support the team's goals and core values can be an easier conversation than criticizing his parenting style.

How can parents help their kid handle heckling?

The only response a player should ever have to heckling is to ignore it. Responding to insults from fans or the opposition only incites further insults. This can be especially difficult for young kids. When they are heckled, they feel that their very self-worth is attacked. Teach them to be as proud of their composure as they are of their skills, and they'll have an easier time.

If a kid is having difficulties with another player on the team, should her parents get involved?

Kids can be brutal. It's in their nature; they're experimenting with the use and abuse of power in a social situation. Sports is one place where we can teach them to do the right thing by their peers.

If your youngster is the one instigating the problem, you have no dilemma to ponder: Tell your child that bullying and/or teasing is not permitted, and ask the coach to discipline your child when it occurs.

If your kid is on the receiving end of bullying from a teammate, there's a real art to discerning what will help her come out stronger. If you think that your child is really being harmed, then you might speak with the coach or the other child's parents. That should put an end to the blatant difficulty, but it won't help your child become a stronger individual, and it may leave underlying tension between your kid and the teammate she's been having difficulty with. If you think your child could handle the situation by standing up for herself, encourage her to do so. There is no better confidence builder than facing down intimidation.

How do you help a youngster learn to stand up for himself against a bully?

How a kid stands up for himself is a large gray area. I believe that the best defense requires composure. Generally speaking, bullies attack those who won't defend themselves. If your child can stand up for herself while maintaining her composure, she stands a good chance of not being bothered again.

You might also consider speaking quietly to the coach about the situation, asking him or her not to interfere in the situation between the two individuals but to work with all the players on team-building. The coach can remind the team that players don't have to be best friends, but once they hit the floor or the field, they are a team, and they must act like it.

If there's an example of bad sportsmanship in a game, what's the best way for parents to address it with their child afterward?

When there's been a dramatic incident of poor sportsmanship during a game, there's often a certain uneasy atmosphere afterward. That's the teaching moment, when you can really capture your kid's attention. Now, before the impact has had time to fade, is a good time to go grab an ice cream with your kid; if you can't do that, talk about the incident in the car while you're driving home.

You might be tempted to open the conversation by asking, "Boy, that was terrible, wasn't it?" Of course you want your child to agree that poor sportsmanship is a terrible thing, but you shouldn't begin by giving him *your* opinion. To get a glimpse of the value system that's building in your child, you have to establish an open dialogue, and the best way to do that is to ask an open-ended question: "Tell me what you think about XXX" or "Why do you think so-and-so did XXXX?"

This kind of teaching moment is transferable to all the events your kid experiences. If through sports you can establish a trend of open dialogue, he'll learn to share with you his thoughts, rather than spitting back what he knows you want to hear. And when it comes time for tougher questions — "I heard that Johnny got busted for drugs at school. What do you think about that?" — you both will be prepared for an honest conversation.

How should parents react when they hear their kid badmouthing his teammates, his coach, or the referee?

Speak up! This is a terrible habit, and the time to stop it is when kids are young. Every kid will at some point say something mean or inappropriate about their teammates, coaches, and referees. When you hear it, that's the teaching moment. Correct it.

- Teammates should be supported, even if they're not your friends.
- Coaches must be respected, even if you don't like the way they treat you.
- Referees are not to be blamed for poor performance; a single call *never* decides a game.

If a kid makes a terrible mistake that ends up losing the game for her team, what can her parents do to make her feel better afterward?

It can be agonizing for a kid — and her parents — when she makes a big mistake, especially if it ends up costing the game for her team. But helping your child regain her spirits and her confidence afterward is a process that has to happen *before* the mistake. Does she have a healthy perspective on winning and losing? Have you modeled a healthy perspective after each of her previous games?

You can't treat every game as a do-or-die situation *except* the one in which your child makes a costly mistake. She'll know that you're just trying to make her feel better, and she won't buy it.

Mistakes are important. Mistakes are what happen when you try to stretch yourself. If you're not making mistakes, you're not trying hard enough. And going through the agony of realizing you have made a terrible mistake can give you a healthy perspective on what it means to try and fail — the sun still came up the next day, you still had to eat breakfast, and eventually it didn't matter quite so much.

If the coach isn't giving a kid the playing time he deserves, what should parents do?

In high school and college sports programs, playing time is an important commodity; if you don't play, nobody hears about you, and you don't move on to the next level. But many parents bring that attitude to the world of youth sports, and it's just not appropriate there. For young kids, being a good teammate is much more important than being an all-star. It's the team-player attitude that is hardest to develop and, thus, should be our first priority to inspire.

If you think your young child isn't getting enough playing time, it may or may not be true. First things first: Step back and take an objective look at the situation. *Why* do you want your child to have more playing time? Does your kid seem upset about the situation, or is it just you?

Is your child getting less playing time because the coach is making a concerted effort to get all players into the game? If that's the case, let the situation be. The coach has established a core value for the team — everybody plays — and is following through on it.

Is your child getting less playing time because the team is enrolled in a highly competitive league and only the best players play? If that's the case, perhaps your child is playing less than other team members because his skills aren't as good. Or perhaps his skills don't complement the coach's game plan for the season. For example, if most of the players on a basketball team are quick, the coach may focus on fast breaks, and in that case, a child who is the best shooter on the team but slow on his feet may not play as much as some of the other kids.

Of course, all the reasons why your child isn't getting the playing time he deserves may be beside the point. If you think your young child is too good to be sitting on the bench as much as he does, think again. If he's really good, he's not going to get any less good by not playing much for a season, provided he continues to practice hard. And sooner or later, this season or the next, with this coach or another, he'll start playing a lot. His teammates will be the ones sitting on the bench. Wouldn't it be great if your child knew how it felt to work hard all season long but still sit on the bench? Wouldn't it be great if he really respected the contribution that the kids on the bench make to the team effort? I've often thought that all kids should experience, at least for a season, what it's like to sit on the bench. It can be a good lesson in humility.

If a kid sits on the bench all season long, how can her parents encourage her enthusiasm for the sport?

This is not the negative situation you might think it is; in fact, it affords parents a remarkable opportunity to connect with their youngster. A kid who sits on the bench will do almost anything to improve — even work with her parents. The first thing to do is sit down with your youngster and talk about setting goals. Then find the time to help her practice. You and your child working together toward a common goal — this is a a nonpressured relationship-building situation that can be filled with moments of connection.

Throughout, be sure to model a proper perspective. The goal should be not more playing time but simply improvement. To keep the youngster motivated, set up concrete ways to measure her improvement.

If a kid is better than most other kids, how can his parents encourage him to be a good teammate?

The opportunity with a star player is to get his value system in order. Now is the time to teach him that with individual talent comes responsibility. In order to do this, parents must model the right attitude when talking with their child: There's a right way to play the game, and it has to do with respect, sacrifice, and being responsible to teammates. Let your young star know, in particular, when you've been impressed with his performance as a team player.

Whether or not your child is a star, you can emphasize to him that truly great players are those who make other players better; great scorers are not necessarily great players. Remind him that kids respect kids who are good — when they are also good teammates.

Should parents encourage their kids to play on elite travel teams and all-star teams?

I strongly believe that travel and all-star teams should *not* be drafted for youth leagues. These kids are much too young to have the "good" players weeded out from the "not-so-good" players. By making this determination at so young an age, we eliminate the potential of late bloomers, throw a wet blanket on the enthusiasm of the "not-so-good" players, and place overwhelming time and emotional pressure on the "good" players. The practice and travel schedules of these young all-stars are insane! Moreover, elite travel teams can really hurt house leagues, often leaving them with too few players and coaches. Even if travel team players are required to participate in the house league, the focus on the travel team often saps the energy and enthusiasm from the house league.

Travel teams are drafted ostensibly to offer young athletes better competition. Good competition is a worthy cause, I admit. But if the quest for good competition involves weekend after weekend after weekend of tournament play, late night and early morning practices, and a win-or-die attitude — all for eight-year-old to twelve-year-old kids, most of whom participate simply because they like sports and have fun hanging out with their friends — are we teaching kids the right priorities? I don't believe so.

Are the problems in youth sports also found in school sports? Are the solutions different?

School programs inherit kids from the youth leagues. They also inherit the problems. In fact, the problems we see in youth leagues often become even more intense in school sports because these programs are more competitive. This is a trickle-up problem, and what we need for that is a trickle-up solution. If we, the adults involved in youth sports, can band together and mold the leagues into the fun, inspiring, teaching experiences that they should be, not only school sports but every element of our communities will benefit.

PHOTO CREDITS

iii Williams College Archives and Special Collections

vi © Aaron Horowitz/CORBIS

viii Williams College Archives and Special Collections

xx Michael Carroll

xxiv Williams College Archives and Special Collections

4 Photo Researchers Inc./Peter Miller

6 © Stock Boston/Martin Rogers

10 © Richard Kalvar/Magnum Photos

14 Williams Sallaz/Duomo Photography

20 © David Wells/the Image Works

26 Billy Hustace/Stockphoto.com

28 © Stock Boston/James Carroll

32 © Steve Warmowski/the Image Works

38 William Sallaz/Duomo Photography

42 © Stock Boston/Bob Daemmrich

47 © Les Stone/the Image Works

50 William Sallaz/Duomo Photography

54 David Roy Bruneau

58 © Mitch Wojnarowicz/the Image Works

60 © Mitch Wojnarowicz/the Image Works

65 David Roy Bruneau

68 David Madison Sports Images, Inc.

69 David Madison Sports Images, Inc.

73 Kathy McLaughlin/the Image Works

76 William Sallaz/Duomo Photography

80 © Stock Boston/David Aronson

86 David Madison Sports Images, Inc.

91 Photo Researchers Inc./Jerry Vachter

98 © Jacksonville Journal Courier/the Image Works

102 AP/WIDE WORLDPHOTOS

108 Paul J. Sutton/Duomo Photography

110 Williams College Archives and Special Collections

119 © Kevin Fleming/CORBIS

123 North Adams Transcript/Chris Dufour

126 Robert Beck/Icon SMI

130 John Mcdonough/Icon SMI

136 © Stock Boston/Jean Claude LeJeune